A PLACE AT THE TABLE

A Place at the Table

Women's Needs and Medicare Reform

Marilyn Moon with Pamela Herd

A Century Foundation Report

The Century Foundation Press ✳ New York

The Century Foundation sponsors and supervises timely analyses of economic policy, foreign affairs, and domestic political issues. Not-for-profit and nonpartisan, it was founded in 1919 and endowed by Edward A. Filene.

LIBRARY OF CONGRESS CATALOGING-IN-PUBLICATION DATA

Moon, Marilyn.
  A place at the table : women's needs and medicare reform / Marilyn Moon with Pamela Herd.
      p. cm.
Includes bibliographical references and index.
  ISBN 0-87078-471-4
  1. Medicare. 2. Women—Health and hygiene—United States. I. Herd, Pamela. II. Title.
  RA412.3 .M66 2002   2002011417

FOREWORD

Buried in the debate about how to finance the retirement needs of Americans are two critical facts: that the overwhelming majority of the elderly are women and that women are disproportionately more likely to be living in poverty in their later years than men. This reality must be taken into account when addressing the structure and reform of programs such as Social Security, Medicare, and Medicaid.

Over the past decade, The Century Foundation developed, sponsored, and published a large body of research and analysis on issues related to the aging of the American population. This emphasis was precipitated by several considerations. Americans are living longer, and birthrates have been in decline. In addition, the aging of the unusually large baby-boom population born between 1936 and 1964 is magnifying the impact of these trends. Finally, the advances in health care over the past several decades have added to the quality and length of life—and to the costs of services, particularly of prescription drugs.

We also were motivated by an increasing concern about the tremendous impact these changes would have on American society and public policy. The inevitable shift of resources required to support the elderly population will not occur without provoking significant political, social, and other tensions. We are continuing our efforts in this area because we have been distressed by the limited scope and value of a great many proposals that have been put forth. In that context, we felt it was important to add balance to the debates that are taking place.

Given these goals, we were delighted to collaborate with Heidi Hartmann of the Institute for Women's Policy Research in finding a new way to approach the issues. After long discussions, we joined with the Institute in reaching out to Marilyn Moon, a senior fellow at the Urban Institute, who is well known for her research and policy analysis in the area of health. For many years, Moon wrote a column on health reform for the *Washington Post,* and she recently completed her term as a public trustee for the Social Security and Medicare trust funds. Pamela Herd, who coauthored the first draft of this report, is a Robert Wood Johnson fellow at the University of Michigan.

In this volume, Moon shows that women are a heterogeneous lot, with varying histories and futures, and she explains why women have different needs from men in terms of their resources and retirement generally. She also shows that the role of women in long-term caregiving is especially important because women actually provide most of such care in the United States. All of these points, she explains, must be taken into account in developing guidelines for policy reform. She then suggests guidelines that would make reforms work for women, including ideas on how to deal with issues such as comprehensiveness, affordability, access to quality care, and the availability of information. Moon concludes that incremental changes are more likely than dramatic restructurings to achieve success.

This report joins the long list of projects in this area that we have supported, including *Medicare Tomorrow: The Report of the Century Foundation Task Force on Medicare Reform;* Joseph White's *False Alarm,* which challenges the conventional wisdom that Medicare and Social Security are in a precarious financial condition; Charles Morris's *Too Much of a Good Thing?,* which looks at how health care spending is valued; two volumes in our Basics series—one looking at Medicare reform, the other at Social Security reform; and two forthcoming volumes, Henry Aaron and Robert Reischauer's new book on Social Security (an update and revision of their earlier *Countdown to Reform)* and Eliot Fishman's *Running in Place: How the Medicaid Model Falls Short, and What to Do about It.*

On behalf of the Trustees of The Century Foundation, I want to thank Marilyn Moon and Pamela Herd for their knowledge and skill in drawing attention to this critical aspect of the issues involved in one of our nation's major programs designed to help older citizens live the last decades of their lives in comfort.

RICHARD C. LEONE, *President*
The Century Foundation
November 2002

CONTENTS

CHAPTER 1

WOMEN AND MEDICARE

Medicare, though designed to serve all elderly, is effectively a woman's program. Women make up three-fifths of all Medicare beneficiaries and an even greater proportion of those who are most vulnerable by reason of advanced age, illness, or low income. Thus, women have the primary stake in how the program functions now and how it may change over time.

This report focuses on women's specific needs and experiences with the Medicare program. Women may face problems that systematically differ from those that men encounter. Part of this analysis concentrates on whether some problems experienced by women are more strongly associated with, say, income or health status, suggesting more encompassing solutions in place of those that would target gender. The ultimate question is: As policymakers seek changes in Medicare over time, how will women be affected?

In theory, Medicare tries to ensure all beneficiaries equal access to a particular set of benefits. The basic benefit package is available to everyone who is eligible for the program. But many circumstances surrounding the lives of older and disabled persons—such as transportation problems, low income, the lack of skilled professionals or facilities in rural areas—affect access to and use of care, causing inequities to arise across different groups in the population. Further, rules and regulations of the Medicare program in practice have impacts on how different groups are treated. Consequently, one important way to assess Medicare's effectiveness is to examine how particular subgroups of the population fare. Do some of these groups—particularly the most vulnerable—face disproportionate barriers to care, intolerable financial burdens, or other problems that suggest ways to improve the program? Will proposed Medicare reforms yield results that are equitable for all these groups?

Basically, women's lower incomes, more widespread chronic care needs, and greater likelihood of either being a caregiver or living alone put them at particular risk with respect to some of the reforms being considered for Medicare. For example, greater emphasis on using private plans to serve this population may add complexity and raise costs for those in poor health. Both as caregivers and as patients, the burdens of decisionmaking about health care choices fall disproportionately on women. Intensifying the inequities, Medicare benefits are not as comprehensive for those with chronic conditions as for other health care needs. Other reforms that are sometimes suggested include a higher age of initial eligibility or greater cost sharing, either of which may be more difficult for women to handle.

A WOMAN'S STEREOTYPICAL LIFE HISTORY

Why are women different than men in terms of their needs and resources in retirement? This is a complicated question that involves people's life histories. Social and economic changes in the past thirty years have begun to put women in living situations more comparable to those of men. But, even if greater equality could be established from this point forward, it would take many years to eliminate the effects of preexisting financial inequities between men and women. That is, differences affecting people in their working years twenty or thirty years ago have a substantial impact on those currently in retirement. Women still have shorter work histories than men and face obstacles to advancement that affect both the level of the Social Security benefits they will receive and their ability to amass pensions and savings.

Although individual life courses are highly varied, there are some patterns that help in understanding why women often end their lives poorer than men and with fewer resources from which to draw to meet their health care needs. Many young women today go on to higher education and enter the labor force in much the same way as men do. But early on, their work histories begin to diverge. Women are more likely to take time out for family and sometimes for caregiving for an older relative. For married couples, it is typically the woman who takes time off and, in many cases, switches to employment that allows more flexibility in hours in order to meet child-rearing demands. And even those women who try to manage more responsible positions may be viewed as being on the "mommy track" anyway. These problems may be compounded for single mothers who bear most or all of the responsibility for raising their children. The usual pattern of divorce is that the woman's living standard falls, while this is seldom the case for the man. Thus, a woman's work history is likely to have some dropout years as well as lower earnings than could be expected for a man engaged in a comparable occupation for each year in the labor force.

The Social Security system, which is the main source of retirement support for many Americans, awards benefits on a formula that uses the top thirty-five years of earnings. A woman entering the labor force at age twenty-two and taking ten years out for child rearing would have to work until age sixty-seven to avoid having her benefit calculated with one or more years of zero earnings. Further, it may be difficult for her to continue working up to retirement age if she does not have a stable work history; employers are not very anxious to hire or retain older workers. If she took lower-paying jobs that offered more flexibility while her children were at home, her benefit also would be lower. If she remained married, she would likely rely on her husband's Social Security benefit; that is, the 50 percent dependent benefit based on his salary might be higher than the benefit she earned on her own. If she divorced after having been married for at least ten years, she would be eligible for a partial dependent benefit from her marriage.

Eligibility for Medicare is somewhat less restrictive. If a woman qualifies for Social Security either on her own or as a dependent of her spouse, even though her work history may be spotty, she will have access to Medicare at age sixty-five. An important caveat, however, is that if her husband retires and receives Medicare at sixty-five, she will not yet be eligible if she is younger. Many women do not realize that they may face a period of being uninsured if their husbands have Medicare but no coverage left over from an employer.

A less consistent work history also means that the typical woman is less likely to have a pension (or that the amount of the pension is likely to be low). Lower earnings over a lifetime, with perhaps the added burden of being a single mother for a substantial part of the working years, translate into lower savings as well in most cases. Thus, a woman on her own entering her retirement years is likely to have fewer economic resources from which to draw. Moreover, many married women depend on the benefits their husbands have earned, such as for retiree pensions or health benefits. A husband's benefits, however, may not always carry over after his death; for example, if a couple opts for worker-only retiree benefits because the dollar amounts of the benefit initially are higher, the woman will be left with much less in the way of financial resources after her husband dies. She may lose access to retiree supplemental health insurance as well, which is important because such insurance affects how much she must spend out of pocket for services that Medicare does not cover.

Women live substantially longer on average than men. Because of this, they are more likely to be the surviving spouse from a marriage, often serving as caregiver at the end of the partner's life. A prolonged illness may drain the family's resources, leaving the widow with fewer financial assets on which to rely at the end of her own life. Moreover, as the survivor, she is likely to need care at some point but will have no spouse to help with that care. Consequently, she is much more likely to have to go to a nursing home to have her needs met than to be able to stay at home. This is not only expensive; it is usually not the preferred choice of anyone who needs substantial care. Reliance on such formal care services is compounded by the fact that women tend to have more frequent incidences of health conditions that stretch out over time. But, as will be discussed later, Medicare does not cover long-term care; the only public program for such services is Medicaid, and its eligibility is restricted to those with low incomes or those who have become impoverished after spending all their resources on long-term care.

Altogether, these issues of concern suggest that women are more likely to rely on Medicare to meet their higher health care needs. And while all Medicare beneficiaries face high out-of-pocket spending on health care, that burden is more onerous for women, with their generally lower incomes.

WOMEN, LABOR FORCE PARTICIPATION, AND RETIREMENT

Although the scenario painted above certainly does not apply to all women, statistics on work and income bear out these claims. Women's labor force participation has increased substantially over time for women of all ages. But at a peak of about 80 percent for those aged twenty-five to fifty-four, participation still remains below the equivalent figure for men, which is closer to 90 percent.[1] Over a lifetime these differential participation rates affect pension accumulations and other critical determinants of women's economic status in retirement.

Women are more likely to have low incomes than are men. Older women tend to have had fewer years in the labor force, so they are less likely to have pensions or savings of their own to help boost their financial status when they live alone. For example, more than one-third of women have ten or more zero-earning years in calculating Social Security benefits as compared to 12 percent of men. At the other end of the scale, three-quarters of men have no "zero" years, while only one-third of women can say the same.[2] Even though women's average benefits are lower, Social Security is still a more reliable source of income than pensions or savings. Women have both fewer pensions and lower values for those pensions as compared to men. Further, lower access to pensions is firmly associated with a lower likelihood of having employer-sponsored retiree health insurance (see Chapter 2).

As Figure 1.1 shows (see page 6), older women are substantially more likely to live in families that have lower incomes than are older men. Many more women are in families with incomes below $15,000, while men's household incomes are more likely to be above $25,000. Six out of ten women are in families with incomes below $25,000 a year.[3] These distinctions become even more stark when we compare nonmarried women's incomes to those of men. The income for a typical unmarried male Medicare beneficiary (measured by the median) was $13,044 in 1999; the typical income for an unmarried woman was 8 percent lower, or $11,999. Keep in mind that women are more likely to live alone: after age seventy-five, nearly 53 percent of women (compared to 22 percent of men) live alone.[4]

Viewed another way, just 6.9 percent of male Medicare beneficiaries had incomes low enough to be categorized as poor, while 11.8 percent of women fell into this category in 1999. Among women age sixty-five and above who live alone, poverty rates reach 20 percent. If the threshold for determining low income is set at 150 percent of poverty (about $13,000 per year), 23 percent of all women—and 44.9 percent of older women living alone—have low incomes.[5]

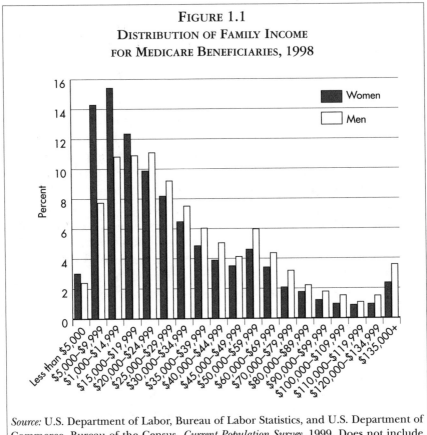

FIGURE 1.1
DISTRIBUTION OF FAMILY INCOME
FOR MEDICARE BENEFICIARIES, 1998

Source: U.S. Department of Labor, Bureau of Labor Statistics, and U.S. Department of Commerce, Bureau of the Census, *Current Population Survey,* 1999. Does not include institutionalized persons.

HEALTH CARE ISSUES

While living longer is desirable, women face challenges during the years in which they outlive men in their cohort. Higher rates of chronic illness and disabilities leave women more vulnerable. Throughout their life course, women are more likely to have chronic conditions that require long periods of medical care.[6] Seventy-three percent of female Medicare beneficiaries have two or more chronic conditions compared to 65 percent of men.[7] Osteoporosis, arthritis, and hypertension are some of the illnesses women are more likely to encounter (see Figure 1.2). They also are more likely to have Alzheimer's disease. A greater chance of living past age eighty-five, at which point illness is more likely to set in for both men and women, accounts for much of this risk. As Table 1.1 shows, while 66 percent of women age sixty-five to seventy-four have two or more chronic conditions, this rises to 85 percent among those eighty-five and over.

Two other measures shown in Table 1.1 (see page 8) indicate even greater differences between men and women.[8] Women's greater propensity toward chronic illness leaves them at a greater risk for disability in old age.[9] Women tend to be disabled for longer periods of time than are men. Men are more likely to improve or die after becoming disabled, while women are more likely to remain the same, worsen, or be institutionalized.[10] In one study, the proportion of disabled women increased from 22 percent of those aged seventy years and older to 81 percent of those aged ninety and over. For men, the comparable statistics were 15 percent and 57 percent, respectively.[11]

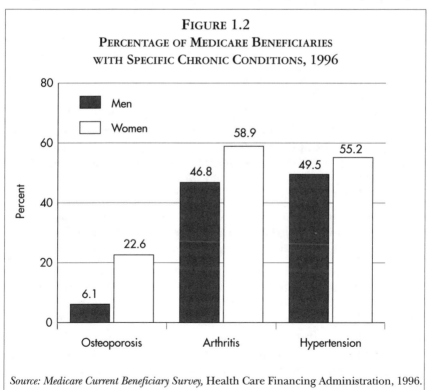

FIGURE 1.2
PERCENTAGE OF MEDICARE BENEFICIARIES
WITH SPECIFIC CHRONIC CONDITIONS, 1996

Source: Medicare Current Beneficiary Survey, Health Care Financing Administration, 1996.

TABLE 1.1

PERCENTAGE OF WOMEN MEDICARE BENEFICIARIES
WITH HEALTH PROBLEMS, BY AGE, 1996

	BELOW AGE 65	65–74	75–84	85+
PERCENTAGE WITH:				
2+ ADL* limitations	70	66	78	85
Severe physical limitations	49	13	28	77
Cognitive problems	50	11	19	54

* Activities of daily living

Source: Authors' calculations from Medicare Current Beneficiary Survey, Health Care Financing Administration, 1996.

Although the disability portion of Medicare (that is, for those under age sixty-five) serves fewer women than men, those who are eligible have comparable levels of disability and require spending similar sums on their behalf.

Quite simply, women are more prone to chronic conditions that leave them with long-term care needs.[12] Disabled women need help with basic activities of daily living like dressing and bathing as well as with what are termed "instrumental" activities, including handling finances, housecleaning, and cooking.

Some of the higher costs associated with disability are for long-term care services not covered by Medicare. Nonetheless, acute care costs rise as well because many disabling conditions stem from medical problems. Since men usually precede their wives in death, women often have no one to provide care for them at home. Consequently, a little more than twice as many female Medicare beneficiaries (1.4 million) are in institutions than male ones. In the case of institutionalization, they may receive help under the Medicaid program. But many women remain in the community, often isolated and in need of supplemental services such as transportation or home health care aides that they may not receive. The problems generated by long-term care needs, both in institutions and in the community, are serious and deserve attention on their own. This analysis, which focuses on Medicare, raises these concerns only peripherally as they are unlikely to be addressed directly by reforms in Medicare. But, in a related issue, many isolated, disabled women may be unable as well to get the acute care services they need.

High out-of-pocket expenses for health care hit women particularly hard because they are more likely to have limited ability to cover these. Women have fewer resources to meet their needs from income, assets, or supplemental insurance. This is particularly a problem as women age. That is, their expenses rise while their sources of financial security decline.

CAREGIVING RESPONSIBILITIES

Despite their greater health problems, particularly the preponderance of long-term care needs, women are more likely to provide unpaid caregiving and less likely to receive it. The majority of long-term care in the United States is provided informally by women.[13] In part this reflects a cultural phenomenon in which women have always been the caregivers in society. Another reason is that men tend to depend on their wives for caregiving, but women are less likely to have that option because of their longevity. At older ages, women are less than half as likely to be married as men,[14] and being unmarried is a good predictor of the need for paid care use simply because there are fewer possibilities for informal care.[15] But even married women are less likely to receive and more likely to give informal care than are married men.[16]

The greater caregiving by women may help to explain what is sometimes called "the marriage effect": married men tend to be in much better health than married women. One study of men and women over the age of sixty-five found that men benefited more from marriage than did women.[17]

Caregiving can threaten women's well-being in several ways. Caregivers have higher rates of depression, sleeplessness, lack of exercise, and drug misuse.[18] They also are more likely to report their health as poor. It is not uncommon, for example, for a woman to become incapacitated following the death of her husband, particularly if she has been the primary caregiver during her spouse's illness. She may have ignored her own care needs while helping him.

Being the surviving spouse can mean a lower standard of living if assets were depleted to pay for an illness or if benefits, such as pensions or retiree health insurance, do not carry over to the widow. Women thus have an important stake not only in their own care but often in that of their husbands. Inadequate access to formal care for men can entail considerable stress on the health of their wives.

HETEROGENEITY

Although there are significant differences between male and female Medicare beneficiaries, the variation across the social strata of women is considerable as well. Differences in income, race, marital status, and health status create large differences in needs. Black and Hispanic women are 50 percent more likely to be in poor health compared to white women. They have more chronic illnesses, mainly diabetes and hypertension, which contribute to higher levels of disability.[19] Black women also tend to have more dire outcomes from the same diseases. For example, although they have lower rates of breast cancer than white women, they are more likely to die from it: 78 percent of white women compared to 63 percent of black women had a five-year survival rate after contracting breast cancer.[20] Black women's mortality rate for cervical cancer is three times that of white women.[21] A black woman's life expectancy is about six years lower than that of a white woman.

Income differences interact with race and ethnicity to create differences in needs for health care. Black and Hispanic women are significantly more likely to be poor (Figure 1.3 indicates the rate of poverty across major racial/ethnic classifications), and it is likely that poverty, even more than differences stemming directly from ethnic or racial characteristics, accounts for their being less healthy in the aggregate than white women.[22] Among all women below the poverty level, 43 percent report fair or poor health, whereas just 20 percent of women with incomes greater than 200 percent of the poverty level say the same.[23] Moreover, minority women are likely to have endured a lifetime of lower incomes and more restrictive access to health care services, helping to explain health status differences from the white majority as they age. These racial and ethnic differences are shown in Figure 1.4.

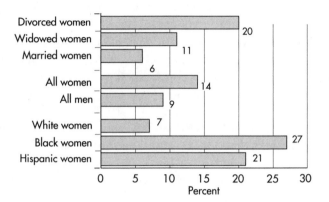

FIGURE 1.3
PERCENTAGE OF MEDICARE BENEFICIARIES BELOW 100 PERCENT OF THE POVERTY LEVEL, BY DEMOGRAPHIC CHARACTERISTICS, 1998

Source: U.S. Department of Labor, Bureau of Labor Statistics, and U.S. Department of Commerce, Bureau of the Census, *Current Population Survey,* 1999. Does not include institutionalized persons.

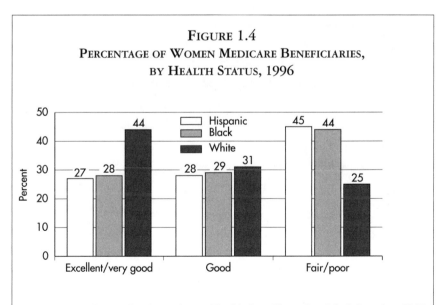

FIGURE 1.4
PERCENTAGE OF WOMEN MEDICARE BENEFICIARIES, BY HEALTH STATUS, 1996

Source: Medicare Current Beneficiary Survey, Health Care Financing Administration, 1996.

The diversity of women's health care needs is evident in their health expenditures. At any given age, a certain segment of the population has more intense needs for diagnosis and treatment and higher costs. This is no different for Medicare beneficiaries. Even among those age eighty-five and over, a small minority account for most health care expenditures each year. Unsurprisingly, the 10 percent of female beneficiaries responsible for the highest spending levels are more likely to have chronic illnesses and functional limitations (see Figure 1.5). This group also bears a greater burden personally. Thirty-nine percent of their income is devoted to their health care expenses, compared to 23 percent for other beneficiaries.

For women, marital status also is strongly correlated with higher income. Marriage provides the man's economic safety net. But when marriages end through divorce or death, women's economic security is threatened.[24] Poverty rates for widowed and divorced women

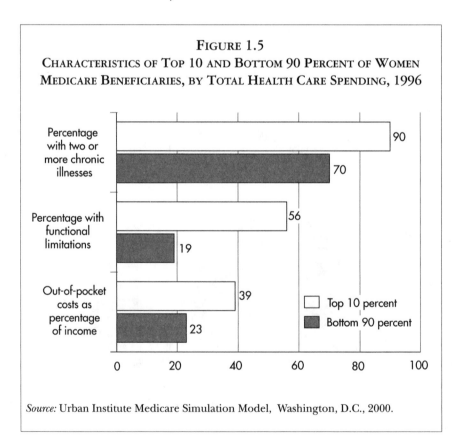

FIGURE 1.5
CHARACTERISTICS OF TOP 10 AND BOTTOM 90 PERCENT OF WOMEN
MEDICARE BENEFICIARIES, BY TOTAL HEALTH CARE SPENDING, 1996

Source: Urban Institute Medicare Simulation Model, Washington, D.C., 2000.

Medicare beneficiaries are about two and three times higher, respectively, than married women's (again, see Figure 1.3). Moreover, women are likely to have fewer assets if they were never married or are widowed or divorced.

A PREVIEW OF REFORM OPTIONS

Despite rhetoric about "protecting Medicare" for beneficiaries, much attention has been devoted to cost-saving measures to slow the rate of growth of what has often been the fastest-rising major part of the federal budget. Some of the enthusiasm for change exhibited in the mid-1990s dulled after the Medicare changes enacted in 1997 as part of the Balanced Budget Act, and efforts to curb fraud and abuse led to dramatically slower rates of growth in Medicare spending at the end of the1990s. For example, Medicare spending actually declined in 1999 even though the program was covering more people. These efforts to slow spending growth proved to be controversial for various reasons, and there have been several subsequent pieces of legislation to mitigate the changes, partially restoring prior levels of payment to many of the providers and private plans that serve Medicare. That revision was made affordable by an economic outlook in 2000 and early 2001 that suggested ample resources in the federal budget to meet a variety of needs.

But times have again changed the outlook. The rapid shrinkage in federal government revenues as a result of recession and new spending demands from the 2001 tax cuts and the September 11 terror attacks have resulted in a bleaker outlook for funding for Medicare. Further, health care costs are now rising faster once more in both the private sector and Medicare, suggesting that cost-saving options soon will be in vogue again.

Reforms under discussion in recent years can generally be slotted into five categories: voucher plans, premium support plans, incremental reforms, changes in eligibility, and expanded financing options. Voucher and premium support plans would result in fundamental changes in Medicare. The philosophy that underlies these major reforms is that competition allows the private sector to be more efficient than the government. Consequently, these approaches would largely shift responsibility for beneficiaries' health care to the

private market and, in so doing, put beneficiaries themselves more at
risk for managing the costs of their care. Incremental approaches
entail more limited changes that maintain Medicare as a govern-
ment-run social insurance program. Private initiatives would still be
used but on a smaller scale. Unlike the first three strategies, which
seek to reduce per capita Medicare spending, the fourth, changes
in eligibility, looks to decrease the number of beneficiaries as a way of
lowering costs of the program. Finally, often in conjunction with
some of the other options, higher beneficiary contributions or general tax increases are sometimes proposed to help meet future needs.

Along with suggestions on how to hold down the growth in
spending on Medicare (to be discussed in Chapter 3), many analysts
and policy makers have raised concerns about the lack of comprehensive benefits in the program. In the 2000 presidential campaign,
both candidates Bush and Gore offered plans for adding a prescription drug benefit, filling one important gap. It is hard to imagine a
"reformed" Medicare program that does not include prescription
drug coverage and a limit on the out-of-pocket costs that any individual beneficiary must pay. Most private plans for younger families
today offer both. While recent attention has focused mainly on prescription drugs, other changes in benefits may be important to consider. But whereas some expansion in Medicare seemed possible in
early 2001, it became more difficult in the wake of the economic
downturn and pressing needs for various defense and security initiatives. Further, the large tax cuts passed in 2001 and scheduled to go
into effect over the next decade will seriously hamper the federal government's ability to find resources for improvements in Medicare. In
the new, less friendly fiscal environment, tax cuts are crowding out other
priorities. The apparent stalemate over drugs in 2002 occurred in large
part over differences in the size and, hence, costs of a drug benefit.

MAKING REFORMS WORK FOR WOMEN

Most of the discussion concerning Medicare reform has focused on
ways to reduce government's commitments, with only lip service paid
to what beneficiaries would want in a reformed program. Protections
for some special groups are raised but are treated as a minor adjustment issue. Yet Medicare was established as a program to help senior

citizens (and later, disabled persons) get access to mainstream medical care, and it is entirely appropriate to assess any reform proposal on the criterion of what would work best for women, who are such a large percentage of the beneficiary pool. Cost issues are valid but must to be balanced with more fundamental concerns about the needs of the people being served.

Medicare's current structure leaves a number of gaps that put all beneficiaries at risk, regardless of gender. While some reforms—such as adding prescription drugs to Medicare—would help, others designed primarily to reduce spending could exacerbate the problems of high relative costs or limited access to care that disproportionately affect women. Thus, five principles will be used to assess the reforms that will be discussed in the concluding chapter:

◆ *Comprehensiveness.* First and foremost is the need to offer comprehensive benefits so that beneficiaries do not have to forgo necessary care. A comprehensive package of benefits would reduce the need for supplemental coverage, which is disproportionately expensive for the very old (eighty-five-plus), of whom 70.7 percent are women.

◆ *Affordability.* Care can only be comprehensive if beneficiaries can afford to pay for the necessary services. Premiums, deductibles, and copayments need to be low enough that it becomes practical for women to use their Medicare benefits. The substantially lower incomes of many older women complicates matters.

◆ *Access to Quality Care.* While an affordable, comprehensive benefit package will help to ensure access to quality care, other arrangements need to be in place. Payments to health care providers by Medicare (or private plans serving this population) must be high enough so that most hospitals and physicians willingly participate in the program. The choice of providers, not insurers, is what most beneficiaries desire.[25] There need to be standards and oversight by Medicare to help maintain the quality of the care delivered, particularly for the very old and frail, who may not be able to play an aggressive role as consumers.

◆ *Stability.* A high proportion of older women suffer from serious conditions that require consistent treatment over long periods and a stable set of health care providers. Studies have shown that the quality of care and its efficiency is improved when patients have a strong, long-term relationship with care providers. Stability in access to those providers is thus a major issue, particularly for women with health care needs that require ongoing attention.

◆ *Simplicity and Information Availability.* Patients always have a need for a straightforward insurance program that they can understand and for credible sources of information to help them participate in decisions about their treatments and choices of plans. The more complicated the system becomes, the more difficult it is for beneficiaries to know their rights within it. For beneficiaries with substantial health problems or cognitive limitations, these goals are even more important. Moreover, traditionally cast as caregivers, women often must see to others' needs as well as their own.

CHAPTER 2

HOW WELL DOES MEDICARE
MEET WOMEN'S NEEDS?

The Medicare program offers basic acute care insurance protection for millions of older and disabled women. No one can be turned down for this coverage, and once it is provided eligibility lasts for the rest of a person's life. Women contribute to Medicare during their working lives, paying payroll taxes that support Part A. When they become eligible, most choose to enroll in Part B, which covers a number of nonhospital services; they pay a subsidized premium for it, with government picking up 75 percent of the costs. It is not surprising, then, that Medicare is one of the most popular of all federal government programs. But it also is a large and complicated program, serving a beneficiary population of nearly 40 million people at a cost in excess of $257 billion in 2002.

When Medicare was instituted in 1966, it revolutionized health care coverage for all persons aged sixty-five and older. It almost immediately doubled the share of seniors covered by health insurance.[1] By 1970, 97 percent of older Americans were covered by the program, and that figure has remained about the same ever since.[2] Most of the focus of legislative debate before Medicare's passage was on what is termed Part A (Hospital Insurance). Hospital stays, skilled nursing facility care, and some home health services are covered by this portion of the program. Hospital care in particular was the major expense faced by seniors. Part B (Supplementary Medical Insurance) was added at the last moment as a program of voluntary participation covering outpatient hospital services, physician services, and other ambulatory care.

This chapter examines both the strengths of the Medicare program and some of the gaps that need to be bridged if it is to continue to meet the needs of its beneficiaries over time. Medicare was created in 1965 as a complement to the Social Security program, and like Social Security it follows a social insurance model. Its benefit package is not very comprehensive, although it has made major contributions in protecting older and disabled women. Some of the increase in life expectancy over the past thirty-seven years can undoubtedly be attributed to Medicare, particularly in light of the fact that improvements in longevity since 1965 have occurred at a faster pace for persons aged sixty-five and over than for the population as a whole. In 1960, women faced a life expectancy at age sixty-five of 15.8 years; by 1998, that figure was up to 19.2 years.[3] This 21.5 percent increase compares to an 8.8 percent increase in life expectancy for women at birth over the same period.

ADVANTAGES OF A SOCIAL INSURANCE MODEL

The basic principles that underpin the Medicare program—universality, redistribution, and pooling of risks—are extremely important in meeting women's broad array of needs that result from generally longer lives, poorer health, and lesser incomes. A Medicare card provides universal access to basic health care services. Once eligible, all Medicare beneficiaries can participate at no cost for Part A and in Part B will owe the same premium. Whereas Social Security benefits are lower for women, who on average have lesser work histories than men, the full value of Medicare is available to them as long as they have a minimum number of work credits or qualify as a dependent of a Social Security beneficiary. This effectively results in a redistribution of protections to those with limited resources. Further, a beneficiary pool spreads the risk and burden of high health care costs across a large group that includes many relatively healthy participants, holding down spending overall and ensuring that care is not unduly expensive for those at risk. This becomes particularly important for the oldest beneficiaries, who are disproportionately women.

UNIVERSALITY AND REDISTRIBUTION

Because Medicare is almost universally available once a woman reaches age sixty-five, it fills in gaps in coverage that many younger women now face. The number of uninsured women aged eighteen to sixty-four rose from 14 to 18 percent between 1993 and 1998.[4] Beyond the uninsured, in 1998 another 8 percent of women did not have coverage at some point during the year.[5] Women may have difficulty accessing health insurance because they are more likely to be out of the workforce caring for children or because they work in jobs that do not offer insurance. When such women do have insurance, they still are more likely to rely on spousal coverage.[6] Because the coverage is not their own, however, they risk losing their employer-subsidized health insurance should they get divorced, for example. There are federal requirements stipulating that employers offer coverage to the former wife of a worker for a period of time, but since she would have to pay the full cost of insurance (with none of the subsidies usually offered workers), it could easily prove unaffordable. But Medicare evens the playing field, guaranteeing insurance to almost one in five women who previously did not have access.

Minority women and those with low incomes are particularly likely to be uninsured before age sixty-five. In 1998, 13 percent of white women, 23 percent of black women, and 42 percent of Hispanic women were uninsured. For women classified as poor, 36 percent had no health insurance. Thirty-one percent of the near poor (defined as having incomes between 100 and 200 percent of the poverty level) lacked coverage.[7]

In addition, the structuring of tax payments into the system allows people with only limited resources to pay little during their working years but to receive the same benefits as higher-income individuals when they become eligible for Medicare. This guarantee of coverage to those who participate earns Medicare the term "social" insurance. It is not just the sharing of health risks but the implicit protections available to all that helps vulnerable beneficiaries—who are disproportionately women. For those with very low incomes, targeted benefits from Medicaid and the Qualified Medicare Beneficiary and related programs fill in some of Medicare's gaps. But one should not discount the value of guaranteeing equal access to a core set of benefits as a means for ensuring that mainstream care will be available.

POOLING RISK

Along with universality and redistribution, another significant advantage is Medicare's large risk pool. Left to the private market, people over age sixty-five would generally not have access to group plans such as those usually offered to workers. Instead, most older Americans would have to purchase individual plans, which do not pull people into a single risk pool. Healthy individuals who are considered good risks would be offered less expensive plans. Those with health problems would pay dearly or in some cases would not be able to buy insurance at any price.[8] Thus, an individual plan fails to spread the risk of poor health and the high costs associated with it. This is not just an issue of poverty because the problem of affordability would extend well into the middle class. When insurance is only available for $5,000 or $6,000 per year, many individuals would have difficulty affording the coverage.

Medicare's pooling of risk is particularly advantageous for women, with their tendency to have more prolonged illnesses and to live longer than men. Women would face a greater risk of not being able to obtain coverage or of being denied coverage the older they got. Medicare guarantees access to health care services for a group who would otherwise face particular difficulties finding coverage in the private market. Compare Medicare to privately provided Medigap supplemental plans, for example. These are plans that individuals purchase to fill in the gaps from Medicare. Most of these plans have substantially higher premiums for people at age eighty-five than at age sixty-five, which is of course particularly disadvantageous for women.

Universality, redistribution, and risk pooling provide millions of American women with insurance that secures access to medical care when they need it the most. By contrast, insurers in the private market face significant incentives to avoid people who are sicker and more expensive to insure. If insurers unilaterally offered insurance to everyone at reasonable rates, they would likely attract the very sick and would quickly lose money. While those in the private market risk losing or failing to obtain coverage as a result of sickness or just getting older, Medicare beneficiaries do not lose eligibility as they age or as their health worsens. It is not reasonable to expect private insurers to accept enrollees who would substantially increase their costs. Indeed, one role of government traditionally has been to make up for the failures of the private sector; this was a strong rationale originally for Congress to pass Medicare legislation, and it continues to justify maintaining the program's promises today.

MEDICARE BASICS

Anyone aged sixty-five or over who is eligible for any type of Social Security benefit (as a worker or a dependent) receives Part A, Medicare's Hospital Insurance, automatically. Persons under the age of sixty-five who have received Social Security Disability Insurance for twenty-four months and persons with end-stage renal disease were added to the program in 1972. Part B, Supplementary Medical Insurance, is voluntary, and anyone with Part A or over the age of sixty-five can join, but individuals must pay a premium to enroll. That premium is $54 per month in 2002. Most beneficiaries do join Part B because the terms are generous, with the government picking up 75 percent of the costs of the coverage.

The Medicare program has continued to grow along with the eligible population. In 2001, about 40 million people—one in seven Americans—participated. Of that total, 23.8 million were women, accounting for nearly 60 percent of all participants. Women dominate the over-sixty-five age group but constitute just 42 percent of disabled beneficiaries who are younger.

THE BENEFIT PACKAGE

When Medicare began, hospital care predominated, accounting for about two-thirds of all spending. But as the nature of care has changed, Part B has become a much larger share of the program (see Figure 2.1, page 22). Care in hospital outpatient departments and in physicians' offices now replaces many surgeries and treatments formerly performed in inpatient settings. In addition, skilled nursing facility care and home health care—referred to as post-acute care—also have increased in importance over time as hospital stays have been shortened. When individuals leave a hospital after only a few days, post-acute care is often needed as a transition, either in a nursing facility or at home with visits from nurses or other skilled technicians. Some of these benefits, particularly home health services, have been used for supportive or long-term care purposes.

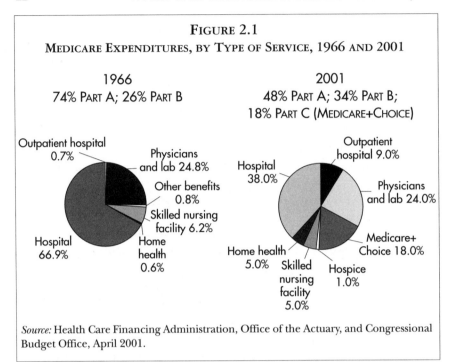

FIGURE 2.1
MEDICARE EXPENDITURES, BY TYPE OF SERVICE, 1966 AND 2001

1966
74% PART A; 26% PART B

2001
48% PART A; 34% PART B;
18% PART C (MEDICARE+CHOICE)

Source: Health Care Financing Administration, Office of the Actuary, and Congressional Budget Office, April 2001.

Women use the services offered in traditional, fee-for-service Medicare differently from men. In particular, as is shown in Figure 2.2, women are substantially more likely to rely on Medicare for post-acute care services than are men. Physician and outpatient services are utilized with similar frequency by both sexes.

Although Medicare's benefit package has changed little since 1965, in terms of how services are provided, the program has kept up with the times. Many surgeries are now performed on an outpatient basis, for example, explaining why the share of Medicare spending in hospital outpatient facilities has gone from less than 1 percent to 9 percent of the program (see Figure 2.1). Today, even the oldest of the old have access to mainstream medical care.[9] New technology is available to beneficiaries, and in some cases the dissemination of new procedures occurs at a faster pace for the old than for the young.[10] Thus, while Medicare today is often criticized for its lack of comprehensiveness, it has given a whole generation of the elderly access to the same basic benefits as younger, healthier beneficiaries, access ranging beyond what they had before. While there is certainly room

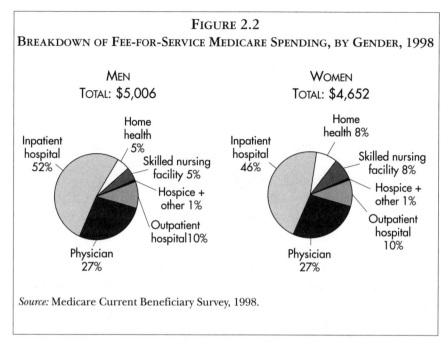

FIGURE 2.2
BREAKDOWN OF FEE-FOR-SERVICE MEDICARE SPENDING, BY GENDER, 1998

MEN
TOTAL: $5,006

Home health 5%
Inpatient hospital 52%
Skilled nursing facility 5%
Hospice + other 1%
Outpatient hospital 10%
Physician 27%

WOMEN
TOTAL: $4,652

Home health 8%
Inpatient hospital 46%
Skilled nursing facility 8%
Hospice + other 1%
Outpatient hospital 10%
Physician 27%

Source: Medicare Current Beneficiary Survey, 1998.

for improvement, Medicare in fact redoubled its commitment to insuring those who are most in need by expanding coverage to persons with disabilities in 1972. Such attributes are particularly important for women, given their vulnerabilities.

TWO TYPES OF COVERAGE

Medicare offers two different types of insurance programs. The first is the traditional fee-for-service program in which the government essentially serves as the insurer. Providers of care for Medicare submit claims, which are processed by firms hired by the government. The federal government bears the risk for the costs of this care. The second Medicare option is now referred to as Medicare+Choice. In this case, the government contracts with private insurers—usually health maintenance organizations (HMOs)—to cover all Medicare benefits for a fixed monthly payment. Beneficiaries then get their Medicare benefits through these private insurance plans, and the plans themselves bear the risk for the costs of care. Medicare+Choice was established in 1997 and replaced the HMO risk option that had been growing as a share of the program since the

1980s. After reaching a high of about 17 percent of beneficiaries, Medicare+Choice enrolled about 14 percent of beneficiaries in 2002.

Initially, the HMO option attracted only a very small share of Medicare beneficiaries because of the restrictions these private plans impose. HMOs require beneficiaries to use only plan-approved doctors and hospitals as a condition of coverage. Beneficiaries in the traditional part of the Medicare program can choose to remain in a fee-for-service arrangement at no extra cost.[11] They are free to use any facility or physician, and almost all providers participate in the Medicare program. Consequently, HMOs need an "edge" to attract beneficiaries. To be more competitive with fee-for-service, many of these plans offer benefits in addition to those covered by Medicare, such as prescription drugs or dental care.

Plans are able to offer more benefits and typically lower cost-sharing requirements in part because of their stricter set of rules for beneficiary participation. In fact, plans are required to provide extra benefits or return money to the federal government if the payments they receive exceed the costs of providing basic Medicare-covered services. The extra benefits and other issues regarding Medicare+Choice are discussed in more detail in the section on supplemental insurance later in this chapter.

BENEFICIARY COST SHARING

Financial burdens on the elderly for health provision fell nearly in half as a result of Medicare's introduction. In 1965, the typical elderly person spent about 19 percent of personal income on health care, dropping to about 11 percent in 1968. Over time, the share of income that seniors spend on health has crept back up (today it is more than 21 percent), but this figure would still be much greater if Medicare were not there (see Figure 2.3). Medicare's contribution to the costs of health care for seniors averaged better than $5,200 per beneficiary in 2000, or nearly one-third of the median income of persons aged sixty-five and older and about half of the median income of women in that age range.

There are several explanations to account for the high level of spending by Medicare beneficiaries themselves. An individual who chooses to enroll in Part B must pay a premium set at 25 percent of the average costs of Part B. Traditional, fee-for-service Medicare also requires individuals to pay portions of their own bills. Both Parts A and B have deductibles, and most of the services are subject to some type of coinsurance. The Part A deductible—$812 in 2002—

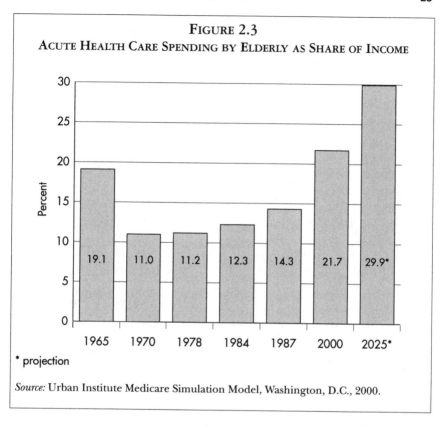

FIGURE 2.3
ACUTE HEALTH CARE SPENDING BY ELDERLY AS SHARE OF INCOME

* projection

Source: Urban Institute Medicare Simulation Model, Washington, D.C., 2000.

is particularly high. And there is no limit on the total amount that any one beneficiary might have to pay. As a consequence, beneficiaries are liable for more than 20 percent of the overall costs of Medicare-covered services. Moreover, as mentioned previously, Medicare is not a very comprehensive program. A number of services, particularly prescription drugs and vision and dental care, are not part of the basic benefit package. Finally, even though many beneficiaries have some supplemental insurance to cover these other expenses, they often pay a substantial amount for such insurance. Together, these additional expenses swell beneficiaries' out-of-pocket costs, which are estimated to have averaged $3,100 in 2000.[12]

FINANCING THE PROGRAM

The Medicare program is basically financed by three revenue sources. Part A relies almost exclusively on a payroll tax of 1.45 percent of wages paid by both workers and employers, resulting in a combined tax rate of 2.9 percent. Part B funding is split, with 25 percent paid in premiums by those who choose to enroll in the program and 75 percent paid out of general revenues (personal and corporate income taxes). Because Part B is becoming a larger share of the program, general tax revenues and premiums are rising as a share of Medicare spending.

Part A, like Social Security, has built up a trust fund that generally gets a lot of attention as one way to focus on the financial health of the program. Its status has varied substantially over time, often coming close to exhaustion. But the good economy of recent years and policy changes have helped, putting off the estimated date of trust fund exhaustion until 2029.[13]

Medicare's strong current financial status should not mask the fact that greater resources will be needed to support this program eventually unless dramatic cuts in eligibility or the generosity of benefits are made. The combination of spiraling costs of care and a doubling of the population on Medicare as the baby boomers retire means that the program's budgetary needs will inevitably go up. In 2001 it was projected that the share of gross domestic product devoted to Medicare would rise from 2.34 percent to 4.51 percent in 2030. Since GDP also will grow substantially over the period, even a larger share going to Medicare may prove to be only a modest burden on society. In all likelihood, increases in both payroll and income taxes will have to be considered to sustain the program. Higher taxes obviously have political and economic consequences.

But the alternative, relying on cost savings extracted from the program, may have adverse impacts on beneficiaries, particularly women. For example, the Balanced Budget Act of 1997 made substantial cuts in payments to hospitals and introduced a new way of paying skilled nursing facilities and home health agencies that is designed to reduce utilization of these services. From the beneficiaries' perspective, some of these changes represented a cut in benefits. Use of home health services (disproportionately by women) declined at the end of the 1990s. Further, a shift of home health care from Part A to Part B, also part of the legislation, resulted in an increase in Part B premiums. While some of the cuts in payments have been moderated by later legislation, more restricted access to services and higher Part B premiums remain as issues for beneficiaries. Changes in Medicare nearly always create hardships for providers, beneficiaries, or taxpayers.

MEDICARE'S GAPS

Despite budgetary and cost concerns, reform discussion also needs to focus on the holes in Medicare's coverage. Medicare alone meets only 50 percent of beneficiaries' health care costs.[14] When Medicare and its benefit package were created in 1965, medical care needs and insurance looked very different than today, and for many workers then it was sufficient just to have hospital coverage. The practice of medicine and the role of insurance has changed considerably in thirty-seven years. Care is more expensive and is delivered differently, and more is covered by insurance for younger workers.

But basic Medicare coverage has remained largely unaltered. As noted above, in areas that Medicare covers, it can and has adjusted to changes in medical practice. But in other areas—such as prescription drugs, which are covered by Medicare only when administered in institutions—changes in care delivery have left Medicare out of step with other insurance plans. One recent study found that 82 percent of employer-based plans had more generous health benefits than does Medicare.[15]

Women are more likely to need prescription drugs and long-term care and are less likely to have access to the comprehensive supplemental coverage that would meet such needs. Consequently, they face particularly high out-of-pocket costs that tax their already limited incomes and threaten their economic security. Women aged eighty-five and above with incomes below $20,000 per year who have serious physical or cognitive handicaps faced out-of-pocket costs estimated at 52 percent of their incomes in 2000.[16]

SUPPLEMENTAL COVERAGE

Because of Medicare's limited benefits, private markets and public programs have developed to meet the additional need for insurance. There are four kinds of supplemental policies. Employer-based retiree insurance and individual supplemental coverage are provided by commercial insurers, while Medicaid subsidizes many low-income beneficiaries. A fourth option is essentially a hybrid: Medicare contracts with private plans, mostly HMOs, to serve beneficiaries who choose to enroll. These supplemental coverage options vary in quality and in the degree to which they relieve financial burdens. Women, it should be noted, may not be able to take advantage of some of the more attractive options because of their work histories (or lack thereof) or financial circumstances. It is difficult to consider how Medicare should change without a good understanding of how these supplemental plans work and of the contributions they make.

EMPLOYER-BASED PLANS. Employer-based plans, to which women typically have less access than men (see Table 2.1), normally offer comprehensive supplemental insurance. Employers usually subsidize the premiums that their retirees are asked to pay and establish benefits comparable to what their working population receives by filling in gaps left by Medicare. A large proportion of these plans, for example, cover prescription drugs. Beneficiaries in these plans have among the lowest out-of-pocket costs, often without suffering limitations on provider choice.[17]

TABLE 2.1
SOURCE OF SUPPLEMENTAL COVERAGE, BY GENDER, 1998

	HMO	EMPLOYER	MEDICAID	MEDIGAP	PUBLIC	NONE
Women	17	32	15	23	4	8
Men	17	37	10	19	4	12

Source: Authors' calculations from *Medicare Current Beneficiary Survey,* Health Care Financing Administration, 1996.

But such generous retiree benefit plans are restricted to workers and dependents whose former employers offer them. As a consequence, these benefits accrue mainly to high-income retirees. It is also important to note that the majority of women who have employer-based coverage have it through a spouse. As Table 2.2 indicates, 64 percent of married women (compared to 16 percent of married men) do not have coverage under their own names. At least some of these married women will lose their employer-based coverage when their spouse dies.

MEDICAID. Medicaid, which also offers generous fill-in benefits to complement Medicare, is targeted toward the poor. Medicaid was established at the same time as Medicare. It is a joint federal/state

TABLE 2.2
PERCENTAGE OF BENEFICIARIES WITH EMPLOYMENT-BASED COVERAGE
COVERED BY A SPOUSE'S EMPLOYMENT-BASED SUPPLEMENTAL POLICY, 1996

	MARRIED	WIDOWED
Women	64	4
Men	16	2

Source: Authors' calculations from Medicare Current Beneficiary Survey, Health Care Financing Administration, 1996.

program in which states have some latitude in establishing eligibility and coverage. Today, four separate programs provide some benefits under the Medicaid umbrella. Basic Medicaid coverage is limited to those with the lowest incomes, generally well below the federal poverty level. For those who are eligible, coverage is comprehensive. In addition to paying the Part B premium and relieving beneficiaries of the responsibility for copayments and deductibles, these state-based programs all offer some type of prescription drug coverage, long-term care, and a range of other services as well.

The remaining programs have been added since 1988 to provide some additional relief for low-income Medicare beneficiaries. The Qualified Medicare Beneficiary Program (QMB) covers Part B premiums, deductibles, and coinsurance for those whose incomes fall below 100 percent of the poverty level (about $8,500 in 2002 for a single person). The Specified Low Income Medicare Beneficiary (SLMB) program covers the Part B premium for those with incomes between 100 and 120 percent of the poverty level but provides no cost-sharing help. Finally, the 1997 Balanced Budget Act created the Qualified Individuals (QI) program to cover the full premium costs for people with incomes between 120 and 135 percent of the poverty level and a small portion of premium costs for those up to 175 percent of the poverty level.[18] Together, these four programs that supplement Medicare are termed the Medicare Savings programs.

In practice, Medicaid and the Medicare Savings programs protect only some of the people who qualify for them. Traditional Medicaid, for example, only covers about half of all persons below the poverty line. Moreover, in 1996, only 55 percent of those eligible

participated in QMB, and just 16 percent of those eligible participated in SLMB.[19]

Women, people of minority backgrounds, and those in poor
health are more likely to rely on public benefits.[20] Table 2.1 shows
that 15 percent of women (just 10 percent of men) rely on Medicaid
or the Medicare Savings programs. These women are likely to be
older and in poorer health than the typical Medicare beneficiary.

MEDICARE+CHOICE. Medicare+Choice (M+C) plans represent
another source of supplemental coverage. The essentials of this
option were described earlier. One big advantage that they offer is
that any premiums they charge on top of the Part B premium tend to
be considerably lower than Medigap rates. An annual premium in
California for AARP's Medigap policy was $893 in 1995 compared
to $117 for risk HMOs.[21] These plans attracted a large number of
new beneficiaries in the 1990s, reaching a peak in 1999 of 7.3 million
beneficiaries.

Private plans can offer extra benefits for two reasons. First, they
usually bring greater efficiency to the delivery of care. In addition,
federal payments to plans historically have been higher than needed
to provide for Medicare-covered services because HMOs enroll, on
average, a healthier pool of beneficiaries.[22] This constitutes an
implicit subsidy from the federal government to the plans. The federal government has not been able to adjust plan payments effectively to account for differences in health status.[23]

The gains from using Medicare+Choice have narrowed since
1998, however, after legislation reduced substantially the growth in
federal payments to plans. By February 2001, after a number of plan
withdrawals from Medicare, their program enrollment had fallen to
5.6 million.[24] For those plans that remain, extra benefits have been
cut back and premiums have increased.

While HMOs have great theoretical promise for coordinating
care that could be particularly helpful for women with chronic conditions, plans have spent more time on seeking discounts than on
coordination.[25] Since they also do better with healthy patients, they
have never sought benficiaries with chronic care needs. Thus, the
private plan option has not fulfilled either of its main promises: to
reduce costs and to be innovative in the management of care. But for
some beneficiaries it remains a source of lower-cost supplemental
insurance.

MEDIGAP. A traditional form of private supplemental coverage, commonly referred to as Medigap, leaves the financing burden resting on the individual. The ten standardized plans that insurance companies are allowed to offer cover a basic package of Medicare's required cost sharing and in some cases include a limited prescription drug benefit.[26] Even the limited drug coverage allowed in Medigap is becoming more difficult to obtain, however. Many insurers have dropped such coverage or have set prices at such a high level that few can afford them. In 1998, only about 500,000 policies were issued.[27]

Such insurance does not, on average, lower costs since the premium, fully paid by the beneficiary, reflects substantial administrative and marketing charges and often profits for the insurer. Thus, many beneficiaries have actually added to their financial burden by buying Medigap insurance. Medigap is most useful for reducing potential catastrophic expenses for those who might have high costs in a particular year. This form of supplemental insurance provides the least protection for beneficiaries, yet it is the most important source of supplemental coverage for women (particularly those of modest means). Women are more likely than men (26 to 22 percent) to rely on Medigap.

Medigap premiums expanded swiftly in the 1990s. Between 1992 and 1996 premium rates in Arizona, Ohio, and Virginia rose 18 percent, 41 percent, and 19 percent respectively, though the bulk of those rate increases took place in 1995 and 1996.[28] National estimates, according to insurance experts, for rate increases in 1999–2000 were in the 8 to 10 percent range.[29] Because of problems of affordability, poor and minority women today are less likely to purchase Medigap plans than they were just a few years ago.[30]

Over time, Medigap plans have changed the way they price policies, which also has made them less accessible. Medigap providers can sell policies that are rated by community, "issue age," or "attained age."[31] In this context, a community-rated premium would be the same for beneficiaries of all ages (and hence work best for women). "Issue age" policies set premiums according to the age at which an individual enrolls. An "attained age" policy allows an insurance company to charge higher rates for older persons, regardless of when they first enrolled. Companies have moved away from community-rated plans.[32] Most providers have gone to an attained-age structure in which policies increase in cost rapidly as people age. This puts greater stresses on women just as their incomes are declining.[33] For the unwary buyer at age sixty-five, these plans appear less costly than community-rated or issue-age options.[34] But, after a six-month period of open enrollment at sixty-five, underwriting makes it difficult for beneficiaries to change Medigap plans. Thus, beneficiaries who choose policies that are inexpensive at first get locked into rising insurance expenses as they age. In some cases, the premiums get to be so high that older women can no longer afford them—just when they need protection most.

NO COVERAGE. Finally, a rising number of beneficiaries cannot afford any supplemental policy. As of 1998, 8 percent of female Medicare enrollees had no policy to cover what Medicare's benefit package does not (Table 2.1). Beneficiaries who cannot afford to purchase supplemental coverage and who are not eligible for Medicaid are among the most vulnerable. High out-of-pocket costs beyond what Medicare covers can prevent them from getting needed care.

The need for supplemental policies dampens the effectiveness of Medicare's universality and redistributive goals. In practice, beneficiaries' access to affordable health care services varies depending on their supplemental policy, and the costs of those policies tend to fall most heavily on those who can least afford it. Burdens on beneficiaries will likely grow larger as new medical technologies further make the Medicare benefit package outdated and inadequate, with the most vulnerable having to choose between the very high costs of supplemental policies or taking no extra coverage at all. Women's reliance on Medigap—which constitutes a relatively unreliable source of protection—may well mean that any crisis in supplemental coverage will strike them first.

THE SPECIAL CASE OF POST-ACUTE CARE AS A LONG-TERM CARE BENEFIT

Medicare's coverage of post-acute care raises issues of particular importance to women. Post-acute care—that is, home health and skilled nursing facility (SNF) benefits—has undergone significant changes over the past twenty years. At times post-acute care has been quite a minimal part of the program, and at other times it has absorbed larger shares of Medicare spending. The history of these policy changes and benefit fluctuations reflects the difficulty of drawing a line where acute care ends and long-term care—explicitly excluded from Medicare benefits—begins.

In strict terms, acute care refers to services beneficiaries receive in hospitals and from physicians for specific medical conditions. Long-term care provides supportive services, such as help with personal needs like eating and bathing, for those with chronic and disabling conditions. The Medicare program's benefits in this area were designed to help beneficiaries recover from acute care events. Often the inability to manage basic activities of daily living is brought on by acute conditions, however. Women have been caught in the struggle to define the limits of what Medicare should provide since they constitute both the majority of beneficiaries with complex acute and long-term care needs and the majority of informal caregivers for these needs. As noted above, the lack of caregivers available to serve their own needs and their modest incomes tend to make women more reliant on public programs. But the lack of explicit long-term care coverage in Medicare leaves a major gap that disproportionately affects women.

The restructuring of Medicare reimbursement methods in 1984 for inpatient hospital care increased the need for post-acute services.[35] That is, earlier hospital discharges generated needs for providing care in other settings.[36] But the government tightened eligibility regulations for post-acute care in the mid-1980s to prevent hospitals from shifting costs to other providers. Consequently, although in the absence of such regulation these services would likely have expanded substantially in response to shorter hospital stays induced by Medicare payment changes, in actuality the rate of growth for skilled nursing facility and home health care did not rise enough to compensate.[37]

Two court cases in the late 1980s led to a relaxation of these requirements, however. As a result of these decisions, post-acute care began its rapid rise in 1989.[38] Home health care, in particular, burgeoned. Between 1988 and 1997 program payments rose from $1.9 billion to $16.7 billion.[39] Home health aide visits, where largely custodial care is provided, constituted the majority of this increase, rising from 34 percent to 48 percent of total home health visits (nurses and rehab specialists) between 1988 and 1997. Critics cite these statistics as evidence that the benefit was increasingly being used to meet long-term care needs as opposed to rehabilitation or other acute care services. Technically, long-term care services are provided publicly only by the joint federal/state Medicaid program and then only to people with low incomes and few assets. Making a clear distinction between acute care needs and long-term care is a difficult call for policymakers looking at both skilled nursing facility and home health care. The growth in post-acute care was filling in an important gap in policy, although that was not its formal purpose. Policymakers who were alarmed at spending trends began to look for ways to slow the growth in home health and skilled nursing care. As a consequence, legislation in 1997 introduced new payment systems for these two benefit areas.[40]

Women, more likely to have illnesses that leave them with functional impairments,[41] are particularly affected by the unstable nature of these benefits. In 1997, 88 men per 1,000 beneficiaries received home health care services, but 122 women per 1,000 beneficiaries received them.[42] Further, as discussed in the previous chapter, women are less likely to receive informal care. Thus, for women with incomes and assets that make them ineligible for benefits under Medicaid, Medicare post-acute care services are the closest they can come to receiving help with long-term care needs.

In addition, women are more likely to *provide* informal care. Consequently, they bear the burden of cuts as unpaid caregivers as well. Many of the home health care services that were limited by the 1997 legislation are likely now being provided by female family members. Supplemental insurance will not pick up the slack since it only fills in for covered benefits. If services are purchased, they would have to come out of pocket. Congress, wittingly or unwittingly, transferred much of the home health care cost to women, both as beneficiaries and informal care providers.

The most vulnerable beneficiaries, women who are black, Hispanic, poor, in poor health, or saddled with functional limitations, are more likely to report difficulties obtaining care in all settings.[43] Consequently, they are most at risk if access is impeded by the new post-acute care payment systems.

THE SPECIAL CASE OF PRESCRIPTION DRUGS

Prescription drugs are the primary acute care benefit excluded from Medicare coverage. Only in the hospital, a nursing home, or a hospice program will Medicare cover drugs (with a few specific exceptions). This lack of coverage is problematic for women because they rely on prescription drugs to a greater extent than men: women average about 20 percent more prescriptions a year than their male counterparts in Medicare.[44]

Part of women's greater use of and higher costs associated with prescription drug coverage is related to their higher rates of chronic illnesses. A 1998 study of 375,000 Medicare recipients revealed that people with chronic health problems have particularly high prescription drug costs.[45] Average drug spending for those with chronic conditions was 50 to 200 percent higher than average spending for the whole sample. That is, women's prescription costs averaged $1,188, while men's were $1,015. Even after adjusting for health status, women's spending is higher than men's. Jan Blustein showed that when comparing men and women who had hypertension, a common chronic condition, women's out-of- pocket expenses for these drugs were $148, relative to $133 for men.[46] And their out-of-pocket prescription costs were about 14 percent higher overall.

Yet women, often making do without private supplemental insurance, are less likely to have their drug expenses covered than men. In 1996, 32 percent of women as opposed to 24 percent of men did not have prescription coverage. Consequently, those without coverage spend more of their own resources and receive 24 percent fewer prescriptions than those who have coverage.[47] Enrollees without coverage spent 83 percent more out of pocket for their prescriptions. And they also were less likely to get needed help; for example, 22 percent of those with high blood pressure who lacked coverage did not purchase any antihypertensive drugs compared to 17 percent of those with coverage.[48] If women had better access to insurance for drugs, the spending gap between men and women might be even greater, as those women who are currently doing without purchased the drugs they need.

In the end, women are hurt more by Medicare's lack of prescription drug coverage and hence would benefit more if such coverage were added. Higher rates of chronic illnesses combined with a lack of supplemental coverage hinders women's access to necessary medications and increases their costs associated with the ones they do receive. Rapidly rising drug prices will only make the issue more pertinent in the coming years. And voluntary private plans are unlikely to fill the gap. Indeed, coverage in this area is eroding as use of drugs is rising.

OUT-OF-POCKET COSTS

Medicare beneficiaries have high out-of-pocket costs that result from Medicare's incomplete benefit package. They vary based on an individual's supplemental policy, health, age, and income. As Table 2.3 (page 36) shows, women's out-of-pocket spending ($2,680) was 15.7 percent higher on average than men's in 1998. And for women below 135 percent of the poverty level, the amount was 26.5 percent higher. Sicker beneficiaries spend more on their medical care and contribute the most toward those costs. Those with at least one activity of daily living limitation, such as bathing or dressing, spent 33 percent of their income toward medical care.[49] As Figure 1.5 demonstrates, the top 10 percent of women beneficiaries by spending are more likely to have chronic illnesses and functional limitations. They spend 39 percent of their income on out-of-pocket expenditures, compared to 23 percent for other beneficiaries.

In the coming years, the rate of income growth for the elderly will not keep pace with rising health care costs. Consequently, even without reforms to Medicare that would increase beneficiary cost sharing, out-of-pocket spending is expected to grow. While a typical elderly beneficiary pays nearly 22 percent of income on health care currently, this figure is projected to rise to 30 percent by 2025.[50]

Low-income beneficiaries, primarily women and minorities, already pay higher out-of-pocket expenses in proportion to their incomes. These segments of the population will be hit hard if the projections are accurate. Those with some type of Medicaid are relatively well protected. But older, low-income women in poor health who do not receive Medicaid already devote about half of their incomes to medical care.[51] The available estimates suggest that beneficiaries have little capacity to absorb new costs, and this fact should be taken into account when considering reforms to Medicare.

TABLE 2.3
AVERAGE OUT-OF-POCKET EXPENDITURES,
BY POVERTY AND GENDER, 1998

	MEN	WOMEN	TOTAL
Less than 135% of poverty level	$1,791	$2,266	$2,106
135%–175% of poverty level	$2,096	$2,694	$2,442
175%–250% of poverty level	$2,360	$2,855	$2,621
250%–400% poverty level	$2,344	$2,835	$2,590
More than 400% of poverty level	$2,316	$2,680	$2,518

Note: Out-of-pocket expenditures also include supplemental premium and Part B premium. Figures also account for 11% underreporting of prescription drugs.

Source: Authors' calculations from Medicare Current Beneficiary Survey, Health Care Financing Administration, 1996.

Indirectly, high out-of-pocket costs can generate another problem for women. The wife is much more likely to be the surviving spouse. And since expenditures on health care are often high in the last year of life, a husband's illness may leave his widow with even fewer resources to meet her own needs.

MEDICARE'S INCREASING COMPLEXITY

Another shortcoming in Medicare relates not to spending on health services but rather to the support that beneficiaries receive from the program. Disseminating clear and credible information is an important responsibility that needs to be improved. The complexity of Medicare's provisions causes considerable confusion that perhaps affects access to care. Vulnerable beneficiaries who face vision, hearing, and other health problems, people with low incomes, and those with low education levels pose special challenges. But even younger, more informed beneficiaries can have problems in dealing with the system. Further, if reforms are instituted that involve greater beneficiary responsibility, for example, in choosing plans, the need for help will be even greater.

Examples abound where the government has failed to provide the necessary information and education for beneficiaries to make good choices. For example, many low-income beneficiaries have not received adequate information regarding their eligibility for Medicaid benefits. Many Medicare recipients who need Medicaid do not get it because of a lack of communication, administrative complexity, and the difficulties they face advocating for themselves. Consequently, full participation by those who are "dually-eligible" is very low.

The Medicare savings programs, which were intended to help low-income Medicare beneficiaries meet cost-sharing needs, provides a specific example of how system complexity translates into beneficiaries' needs not being met.[52] Twenty-seven states process Medicare savings program applications only at state or county welfare offices, while beneficiaries apply for Medicare at their local Social Security Administration office. The application forms for these low-income programs can be up to six pages long, with complicated directions and small print. It can take from one to six months and in extreme cases up to seven years to activate the benefit. As a result, the program covers less than half of those who qualify.[53]

All beneficiaries need better, clearer information about their options in deciding between HMOs and Medigap and in making choices within the HMO market.[54] One study of more than 1,600 Medicare beneficiaries found their understanding of HMOs to be woefully inadequate.[55] Thirty-one percent of beneficiaries in markets where they had access to numerous HMOs knew almost nothing about them. Beneficiaries in HMOs actually knew less about them than those enrolled in traditional Medicare. For example, only 63 percent of HMO beneficiaries knew they had a right to appeal denial of care. Information disparities between HMO providers and Medicare beneficiaries have led to unfortunate incidents for enrollees. Some HMOs provide incomplete details to beneficiaries, emphasizing their extra benefits but not disclosing the limited provider choice. An analysis of Medicare HMO ads showed that a number of companies incorrectly stated they did not accept those under the age of sixty-five.[56] HMOs are not allowed to deny disabled beneficiaries coverage, but they may imply that such coverage is not available.

Women, by virtue of being greater consumers of care in their old age and being the traditional caregivers, are likely to risk disproportionately high costs stemming from this complexity and lack of information. While not technically a "gap" in Medicare coverage, the consequences of these administrative problems can be less access to care. Thus, this issue needs to be taken seriously.

CHAPTER 3

CONSIDERING WOMEN'S NEEDS
IN REFORM DEBATES

Discussions concerning Medicare reform can center on improvements to the range and reach of services the program provides or on efforts to slow spending growth. Clearly, these goals are not always consistent. Chapter 2 examined a number of short-comings in the current program's offerings. But many policymakers are primarily intent on promoting efficiency or creating limitations in Medicare's scope that will obviate or reduce the need for new tax revenues. To see how the tension between service enhancement and savings efforts is manifested, witness the efforts of the Bush administration and a number of members of Congress to link any proposed expansion of prescription drug coverage to other, less popular changes such as requiring beneficiaries to choose private plans or pay more for traditional Medicare. While reforms that are meant primarily to rein in government outlays are often debated in abstract terms emphasizing projected spending over time or analyzing the incentives that such reforms are intended to establish, this chapter takes a different approach, looking at reform options in light of how they will positively or adversely affect women in practice. One of the great challenges in revamping Medicare is making sure that any reform does not result in the program abandoning the principles that serve to protect many women.

WHY IS REFORM ON THE AGENDA?

Although in many ways Medicare has been one of the most successful federal programs of recent decades, it has faced substantial criticism for its rapid budgetary growth over time. At $241 billion in spending in 2001, it represents about 12 percent of federal government expenditures. Either new revenues will have to be found to support Medicare or its growth will have to be curtailed. Much of the concern about the future is driven by the expected increase in the numbers eligible for Medicare, from 40 million in 2001 to 78 million in 2030, when the entire baby-boom generation will have reached retirement age. While the numbers covered by Medicare have already doubled since 1966, this next doubling of the population will be more significant because the share of the Medicare-eligible population also will grow, from one in every seven Americans to more than one in every five. Women will continue to represent more than 60 percent of the population on Medicare.

Supporters of Medicare would prefer a boost in revenues to continue the success of the program. Since 1965, Medicare has expanded its coverage from 19 million to 39 million people, and its costs have grown at a per capita rate that is less than the equivalent rates of private insurance since 1970. It accepts all eligible persons with no underwriting, charges premiums that are the same for all Part B beneficiaries, and has adapted to many changes in our health care system over time. During its existence, the life expectancy of older Americans has grown faster than for other segments of our population. And, although its benefit package has lagged behind the times, it is still the most important source of health care support for one in every seven Americans.

Recently, the concern for preventing the program from becoming too large a share of the nation's resources has diminished in urgency because the outlook for Medicare's future has improved. Changes made in Medicare by the Balanced Budget Act of 1997 and a strong economy through early 2001 pushed the projected hard times further into the future. The economic downturn of 2001–02 will likely again raise concerns about spending levels, although the 2002 projections continue to look strong. Over time, Medicare's costs will still rise substantially on a per capita basis because new technology and treatments are likely to continue both to cost more and to improve the health and quite possibly extend the lives of those receiving such care. Thus, a legitimate concern is to what extent it is desirable to drive spending lower and, if so, by how much? From another perspective, it is important to question whether we as a society value such benefits enough to consider adding more public money as at least part of the solution. Strengthening the adequacy of benefits would require an even greater commitment of resources.

Restructuring the Medicare program will be a major challenge for some time to come, in part because it is politically easier to propose such changes than to discuss how to raise new revenues. Proposals for restructuring are driven by their perceived effectiveness in holding down the costs of care, although the claims are theoretical at this point. What evidence there is suggests that few savings will arise unless costs are shifted onto beneficiaries. Another issue raised by some policymakers is a desire to have the government play a smaller role in Medicare and to stress personal responsibility by individuals for the costs of their own care. This argument often emphasizes the heavily regulatory nature of Medicare. The appeal of a private approach has colored the debate over Medicare's future for several years.

But this debate can ignore individuals' stake in the process. What about concerns for the goals described in Chapter 1 for evaluating reforms? Affordability, quality, stability, and simplicity all need to be examined. Moreover, for women, at this aggregate level, the issue comes down to a sense of intergenerational and redistributional justice. How much does society want to spread the burdens of care for persons of advanced age and disability? Women's longer lives and lower resources suggest that they will suffer disproportionately if this sense of shared commitment diminishes.

REFORM OPTIONS INTENDED TO GENERATE SAVINGS

The most complicated debate on reform is likely to take place around the role for private insurance in covering Medicare beneficiaries and what that means for traditional, fee-for-service Medicare. Other options include proposals to restrict eligibility or raise beneficiary contributions.

THE RANGE OF POSSIBILITIES FOR PRIVATE PLAN PARTICIPATION

Proposals for reform range across a continuum of how much to rely on private insurers to provide services for Medicare beneficiaries. The most dramatic option would be to establish vouchers for health care, a system in which Medicare beneficiaries would be given a certificate to be presented to a private insurer of the beneficiary's choosing. This voucher would pay a set amount for insurance, usually based on overall average costs and with some likely adjustments to payment level to reflect health status, age, or other indicators of high risk. If individuals choose an inexpensive plan, then they will not pay very much in addition—assuming the voucher is adequate for a basic plan. At the other end of the continuum would be a return to traditional Medicare, with no options for private plans. This would simplify the program substantially. But it also would mean that no HMOs or other private options would be available to those who prefer that type of arrangement.

In practice, only a small group of people advocate a pure voucher setup, and elimination of private plans is not being seriously discussed. Rather, the range of possibilities envisions a mixed system with greater or lesser reliance on private plans. But the details of these proposals are important, and it is certainly possible that, if poorly designed, the system could move further to an extreme than is envisioned by supporters of particular options. For example, if the emphasis is on traditional Medicare and private plans continue to leave the market, most beneficiaries would have little or no choice of plans. On the other hand, without good adjusters for differences in health status and other active oversight by government, an approach relying substantially on the private sector might effectively become a voucher system, with traditional Medicare disappearing as an option. Traditional Medicare could simply become too expensive for most beneficiaries if it continued to attract a sicker than average beneficiary population.

THE ROLE OF PRIVATE INSURANCE AND MEDICARE

A mixed system retaining traditional Medicare and expanding the role for private plans could be achieved gradually using an incremental approach, as will be described below. But a more commonly debated proposal is to "restructure" Medicare to directly rely on competition. This approach is referred to as "premium support."

The goal of premium support is to encourage beneficiaries to choose plans that offer good value in terms of both price and quality. That is, this approach would require beneficiaries who choose more expensive plans to pay higher premiums to enroll. This is quite different than the current system, in which Part B premiums do not vary regardless of whether beneficiaries choose fee-for-service or private plans. The usual proposed structure of premium support is for government to pay to private plans a set dollar amount that represents, say, 80 percent of the costs of an average plan. In that way, some beneficiaries would pay little or nothing if they chose less expensive plans, while others would have higher premiums. Making beneficiaries sensitive to the costs of health care should encourage plans to compete on the basis of price of the premium. This is a more modest approach than using vouchers, although the philosophy is much the same: beneficiaries need to be responsible for helping to hold down the costs of care. Beneficiaries would presumably respond by shifting to less expensive or higher-quality plans when allowed to choose each year.

Practically speaking, would these incentives work as planned? Studies of participants in California's health plan for state workers and in the Federal Employees Health Benefits Program have shown that healthy, young workers respond to market signals as predicted, but retirees resist shifting plans in response to changes in the level of the premium.[1] This is probably a reasonable response by retirees, who are more likely to have health problems already or even to be in the middle of a course of treatment. Switching plans in those situations would not only be inconvenient; changing doctors and other providers that are familiar with an individual's care might not be good for his or her health.[2]

Given the opportunity, the sickest and poorest beneficiaries are likely to remain in fee-for-service Medicare disproportionately—just as they do now—creating substantial challenges for this component of the program. People with severe medical problems—both physical and cognitive—are more likely to have two or more physicians on whom they rely and may find it difficult or undesirable to move to a new system. As shown in Figure 3.1 (page 44), more than one-third of women who currently remain in fee-for-service have such physical or cognitive problems that could affect their desire to switch to a private health plan. The proportion is nearly the same for men, but spending on behalf of women with major medical problems is particularly high, accounting for nearly two-thirds of the spending by all women in traditional Medicare. If these women remain in traditional Medicare, it will become more expensive relative to private plans. If government payments to plans can be appropriately adjusted for differences in health status, this approach may work. Without such adjustments, the most vulnerable women would face sharp increases in premiums to stay in fee-for-service. The same problem could arise for a private plan that attracts and retains a sicker than average population unless it was possible to fine-tune adjustments to prevent it.

The usual defense of a "choice of plans" approach is to simply assert that payments from Medicare will be adjusted for health status. Considerable work still needs to be done on improving such risk-adjustment

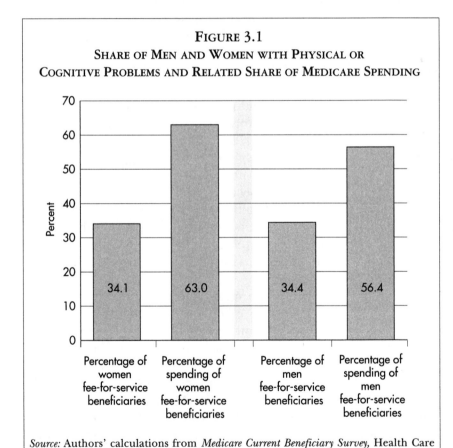

FIGURE 3.1
SHARE OF MEN AND WOMEN WITH PHYSICAL OR
COGNITIVE PROBLEMS AND RELATED SHARE OF MEDICARE SPENDING

Source: Authors' calculations from *Medicare Current Beneficiary Survey,* Health Care Financing Administration, 1997.

mechanisms, however, so that plans have incentives to treat sicker beneficiaries. Thus far, private plans have resisted greater reliance on risk adjustment, and even experts often question whether the tools at hand are sufficient to move quickly toward more extensive participation by private plans.

Until reliable adjustment mechanisms are implemented, private plans will strive to attract healthier than average beneficiaries. Consider, for example, the ads these plans use: they are more likely to show seniors playing tennis than someone in a wheelchair.[3] Since women with chronic diseases are known to be expensive patients, they will not be encouraged to join private plans. This means that extra services offered by commercial plans will not be in areas—such as extended home health benefits—that would entice those with chronic conditions. Ultimately, the sick may only be welcomed in fee-for-service Medicare. As a consequence, for the indefinite future, the bulk of Medicare dollars will be spent in traditional Medicare, an area that is often ignored while the attention of reformers is focused on promoting private plans.

Incremental approaches are less well defined than the premium support proposal. They may lead in the same direction but at a slower pace and with more protections for traditional, fee-for-service Medicare. If the basic structure of the Medicare program is kept intact, there is still a wide range of ways in which the program could be altered to improve its prospects for generating some additional savings. The goal is to make practical adjustments as problems arise rather than starting over with a whole new system. For example, the Medicare+Choice program needs to develop a new way of compensating private insurers. So far progress has been slow in this area for reasons discussed earlier. Moreover, demonstration models that would consider competitive bidding procedures have failed for a range of reasons including active opposition from HMOs.[4] An improved payment system is critical for the success of any arrangement that includes choice of private plans. One advantage of incrementalism is to allow more time to experiment in order to get the payment structure right before requiring all beneficiaries to participate.

Improvements in the oversight of benefits covered by Medicare could also help control expenses in the fee-for-service side of the program. Some innovations in managed care involve coordination tactics that Medicare might be able to adopt. For example, traditional Medicare could offer help to manage treatment of diseases that require careful balancing of providers and procedures. Women, with their higher incidence of long-term conditions, are particularly likely to benefit from disease management and other coordination activities. While Medicare may not be able to institute the types of restrictive controls that some HMOs use to ration services and hence would save less, some limitations can nonetheless be devised. But if not carefully done, efforts to limit utilization in fee-for-service care could put women at a disadvantage, for example, if changes instituted are similar to the new post-acute care payment systems that result in incentives to skimp on treatment and support services, particularly at the high-use end. Arbitrary changes are likely to be easier to implement than true coordination of care used by aggressive managed care organizations. As is frequently the case, the devil is in the details. But for women, the desirability of changes in fee-for-service Medicare will likely turn on whether reforms improve care through greater efficiencies in treatments for chronic illness or disability or whether they simply achieve savings through cutbacks without much regard for quality of care delivery.

Another criticism lobbed at traditional Medicare is that the combination of a fee-for-service system and nearly first-dollar supplemental coverage (that is, minimizing cost sharing) encourages overuse of services.[5] Those with supplemental insurance use one-fourth to one-third more services than those without policies.[6] Yet going without supplemental coverage means exposure to the very high cost sharing that Medicare requires. One way to restructure incentives for beneficiaries to address this objection would be to expand Medicare's basic benefits enough to discourage purchase of supplemental benefits while still keeping some cost sharing in place. The basic Medicare program could be changed to look more like the insurance plans that many workers now hold. Cost sharing would be reduced in amount, and upper-bound protections from extraordinary expenses would be added. Alternatively, private Medigap policies could be restructured to encourage cost consciousness by adopting a similar approach, although this would only affect a subset of supplemental policies. (Employer-provided benefits, for example, could still be used to obtain first-dollar coverage.) Under either strategy, it would be important to keep cost sharing at a reasonable level so that it would not hinder access to needed services. Making changes in Medicare would be particularly advantageous for women since Medigap policies are seldom a good deal for the very old.

The trade-offs between stopping unnecessary service use and stinting on necessary care need to be carefully assessed if the benefit structure is changed. Policymakers need to guard against retooling copayments in a way that would force beneficiaries to be so cost conscious that they undermine their own health, postponing or doing without needed care.

PRINCIPLES TO EVALUATE REFORM PROPOSALS FROM A BENEFICIARY'S PERSPECTIVE

Although reforms to restructure the Medicare program are offered as a means for generating budgetary savings, with the presumed additional advantage of giving patients more choice, these are not the only issues that ought to be considered. Health policy specialists need to keep in mind society's goals in establishing Medicare and to take note of the improvements that many beneficiaries would like to see; these considerations ought to be part of the debate.

SOCIAL INSURANCE. The broad social goals of Medicare, including universal coverage, redistribution of the costs of insurance to protect those with limited resources, and risk pooling to ensure protection of the most vulnerable, have served women well over the years. But these seem almost to be secondary concerns in the minds of those stressing savings and private plan initiatives. Private insurers by design are interested in satisfying their own customers and generating profits for stockholders. Their plans cannot be expected to meet larger social goals such as making sure that the sickest beneficiaries get high-quality care. Consequently, additional safeguards would have to be added to a premium support approach to balance these concerns. While that is certainly possible, such measures add complications to the program and can reduce its flexibility. They also entail a strong role for government, something many premium support advocates would resist.

Women's generally more vulnerable status in society makes them particularly likely to need the protections implicit in a social insurance framework. They have a stake in government's playing a strong role to ensure that these principles are not eroded.

COMPREHENSIVENESS. The structure of the Medicare program (whether it relies on private plans or more on traditional fee-for-service

Medicare) does not necessarily affect its comprehensiveness. Benefits *could* be expanded under either general approach. And although some proponents of private plans have suggested that they would naturally offer superior benefits, one only has to look at Medicare+Choice with its shrinking benefit packages to realize that this is not necessarily the case. The voluntary offering of extra benefits by private plans can attract sicker beneficiaries, and benefits such as prescription drugs are expensive. As a result, as government payments to private plans have grown only slowly, plans have responded by reducing the comprehensiveness of their benefit packages over the past four years.[7] Comprehensiveness depends on a willingness on the part of either beneficiaries themselves or taxpayers to put more resources into the program. For benefits to be guaranteed over time, they need to be made part of the program's basic package. As noted above, women's use of prescription drugs is very high, and adding a drug benefit to Medicare would be especially helpful to them.

Comprehensiveness also depends in part on the controls that private plans may put on access to various types of services. Very strict HMOs usually not only limit patients to seeing providers on a specific list but also may require prior permission to see specialists or have certain tests or procedures done. There are many high-quality HMOs that do this responsibly, with patients' interests in mind as much as managing costs. Other HMOs, however, have proved to be more arbitrary in their demands on patients, compromising access to care. One concern about a system based on the goal of eliciting strong competition through offering low premiums is that the less expensive plans may be the very ones with these arbitrary limits. This is likely to be particularly important for post-acute care, where there are fewer norms and standards to use to hold plans accountable. Anecdotal evidence suggests that HMOs have been markedly restrictive in the area of home health care, which is a service used primarily by women.

AFFORDABILITY. Traditional Medicare poses affordability problems because it compels beneficiaries to share in paying for certain vital services. The costs of supplemental policies meanwhile are rising even faster than Medicare itself, which puts many women in a difficult position. If a more comprehensive benefit were offered under any alternative structure for Medicare and at least partially subsidized by taxpayer contributions, affordability would no longer be such a major concern.

Private plans can offer a better deal for any given package of benefits *if* competition holds down the costs of care overall and slows the growth in premiums and associated costs. Managed care plans often replace required payments by beneficiaries with other controls on the use of services. In the 1990s, the appeal of the Medicare HMO option was that plans were able to offer beneficiaries extra services either at no additional cost or at a premium well below Medigap price levels. The policy problem is sorting out whether that happened because Medicare payments to private plans have been too high, effectively giving insurers an unneeded subsidy to offer benefits beyond traditional Medicare that they would have made available in any case, or whether private plans truly are more efficient. As discussed previously, it is not clear that these plans can be substantially less expensive than Medicare if they have the same mix of sick and healthy enrollees as the traditional program. Private plans may find savings from greater efficiencies, but they must first offset the costs of a substantially higher administrative burden than traditional Medicare carries.

Even if private plans can prove that they can be less expensive, traditional Medicare will be the "default" plan for many years. Some beneficiaries with substantial health problems will view private plans as unrealistic options. Older women may simply be reluctant to adjust to a new system of care. Withdrawals of plans from various locations have created a less stable benefit for many than traditional Medicare. Further, private plans may not be available to people in rural areas. Thus, regardless of the efficacy of private sector alternatives, there needs to be a strong public commitment to protecting the affordability of traditional Medicare for vulnerable beneficiaries. Premium support reforms that put traditional Medicare at a disadvantage will be viewed as undesirable from the standpoint of many older women.

QUALITY OF CARE. In discussing reforms meant to achieve savings for the federal government, the question of whether price competition will win out over quality of care is of considerable concern. Studies of employers' behavior suggest that they mainly choose plans on the basis of price, without much regard for quality. Insurers, then, face incentives to focus on price at the expense of securing the best skilled professional care possible (which may raise costs somewhat). If the government took the same approach in dealing with private plans, women could face hard choices about cost versus quality, particularly since women would be less able to choose higher-cost plans.

Another concern in this area is oversight. Advocates of less government interference and regulation run the risk of de-emphasizing quality. Who will hold plans accountable, and how will they do this? This is also an issue in traditional Medicare, although individuals are able to vote with their feet if they do not like the care they are receiving from a particular provider. This "provider shopping" probably raises the costs of care, but until better information is available to beneficiaries, they will continue to engage in such behavior. Which is more acceptable: provider shopping in traditional Medicare or the tighter controls preventing this in private plans? The answer depends on whether the goal of the overseer is price or quality. But it also depends on whether we as a society continue to make progress on measuring quality and appropriateness (that is, the effectiveness of particular treatments and procedures) and on how well private plans do in coordinating care. Such coordination can lead to quality improvements if it steers patients in the right directions. As yet, the jury is out on how many private plans do this.

Finally, levels of payments to doctors, hospitals, and other providers are an important quality issue. If those payments get to be too low in either traditional Medicare or private plans, participation of providers will go down and patient choice and access will suffer. Traditional Medicare relies heavily on holding the line on reimbursement to hospitals, physicians, and other health specialists as a way to keep in check the costs of care. While HMOs have the ability to impose a broader range of controls, they too lean heavily on keeping reimbursements low. It is difficult to make comparisons between private plans and Medicare at this point in time because much of the information about payments to providers by private plans is proprietary. But what private plans do clearly matters in the deliberations over reform options that could affect quality of and access to care.

STABILITY. Changing doctors or other health care providers or learning new rules concerning insurance is annoying to healthy individuals and disruptive for the sick, who may be dependent on a wide group of professionals to provide their care. Thus, a desire for stable insurance coverage is natural, and this is particularly important for women as they age. Traditional Medicare is likely to have an unambiguous advantage over private plans in this respect. Because nearly all doctors, hospitals, and other suppliers of care services participate in the Medicare program, most beneficiaries do not have to worry about changes from year to year.

When a Medicare beneficiary chooses a private plan, that plan obligates itself to participating in Medicare for only one year at a time. In January 2001, 934,000 beneficiaries had to find new arrangements when their managed care plans decided not to continue in the program. This meant joining another HMO with new rules and new lists of providers or returning to traditional Medicare and negotiating for new supplemental coverage. Not only do participants who decide to enroll in HMOs need to make adjustments initially, they do not have any assurance that the plans will stay with Medicare or that the special benefits that first induced them to enroll will remain the same over time.

Improvements in Medicare+Choice or a whole new private plan system could reduce such disruptions, but the nature of competition is that new plans will come into a market and others, who find they are not competitive, will leave. Withdrawals should be expected; indeed, they are a natural part of the process of weeding out uncompetitive plans that cannot attract enough enrollees or establish good provider networks. Stability can be improved but never guaranteed unless we choose as a society to overpay plans vastly as a bribe to keep them in business. That runs counter to the reason for relying on competition.

Another stability concern relates to plans' contracts with care providers. Patients may join an HMO in January, for example, because their doctor is in that plan. But the doctor or the plan may terminate that contract during the year, leaving beneficiaries stranded without access to that physician unless they go out of network and pay on their own for care. Again, traditional Medicare seldom faces this problem.

SIMPLICITY AND INFORMATION. Women's longer lives, lower incomes, poorer health, and more limited education make it harder for them to be strong consumers and protect themselves in the market. Yet they are often responsible not only for themselves but for spouses in poor health as well. In truth, even people under age sixty-five and of sound mind have difficulties navigating the health care market. Inadequate information, complicated administrative structures, and the market's overriding profit motive provide powerful arguments for maintaining a strong government role in Medicare to protect consumers and their health. In order for a premium support model to meet these needs, considerable investment in accountability, and oversight of private plans would be required—even more than what is needed under the current system, which allows some plan choice. The very nature of adding a layer of required choice of plans to the system suggests that complexity would increase. Perhaps the most disadvantaged beneficiaries in this case are older women living alone and quite possibly isolated from the types of support needed to help them make such decisions.

A good managed care plan that puts resources into support and information could simplify care for many beneficiaries. That is, if doctors worked together truly to coordinate care, the benefits to a sick and frail population would be substantial. PACE (Program of All-Inclusive Care for the Elderly), for example, offers such a model for those who are very frail and otherwise likely to be in a nursing home. But at present it only serves about eight thousand Medicare beneficiaries, and there are few other strong models from which to conclude that the promise of better care will be met by private plans.

Finally, the low-income protections afforded to Medicare beneficiaries by Medicaid and the Medicare savings programs already require long and involved applications; coordination across states and private plans would further complicate the process for beneficiaries in a premium support model. Would all plans take the "dual eligibles," and, if so, what extra benefits would be available and would states have additional requirements?

IMPROVED BENEFITS

It is hard to imagine a "reformed" Medicare program that does not tackle the two vital issues of coverage of prescription drugs and limits on the out-of-pocket costs that any individual beneficiary must pay. When Medicare was passed in 1965, the benefit package was reasonable as compared to available private insurance. But, over time, private insurance has added to what is covered, while Medicare has changed little.

Expansion of Medicare's basic benefit package would be expensive, which has discouraged realization of the many efforts to add benefits over the years. But a more critical stage has been reached because the supplemental plans that have filled in gaps from Medicare also are in crisis, as described in Chapter 2. Private supplemental (Medigap) plans are becoming unaffordable for average-income beneficiaries. Costs of policies have risen rapidly as those who buy plans tend to have greater health problems.[8] Medigap plans are most expensive for those beneficiaries least able to afford them, the very old—disproportionately women. Further, both HMOs and employer-subsidized insurance plans are pulling back on the benefits they offer. Thus, beneficiaries have fewer ways to supplement their Medicare.

A more rational Medicare benefit package by itself (not including drug coverage) would not have to be extraordinarily expensive. Medicare could increase cost sharing in areas such as raising the low Part B deductible while reducing the unusually high hospital deductible and adding protection for those with very high expenses ("stop-loss").[9] This is likely to be an important element of incremental reforms that envision modification of the traditional program to encourage less reliance on supplemental plans over time. A barrier to such changes, however, is political: protections for high expenses help only a few people at a time but generally are paid for with increases in premiums or cost sharing that affect many more. Although insurance is supposed to assist those with high expenses—on the theory that this could happen to anyone—many analysts focus only on a short time horizon in determining winners and losers from such a policy change. This causes good ideas to be abandoned before they can be put in place.

Prescription drugs are not only an increasingly important part of health care but also one benefit that is expensive now and expected to grow more so over time. Those purchasing Medigap plans can at best obtain limited prescription drug protection. (Increasingly many private managed care plans also restrict these benefits.) Drugs pose a potent risk selection hazard; private plans that offer prescription drug benefits find that they attract sicker patients. The response has been for HMOs to restrict this coverage by putting a limit on what they will pay and for Medigap policies to raise prices substantially for a specified drug benefit. In order to ensure future availability of prescription drugs, they must be integrated into an expanded benefit package regardless of whether premium support or incremental reforms are the preferred approach.

As pointed out in Chapter 2, women who lack coverage for drugs use fewer of them, likely skimping on necessary as well as more dispensable prescriptions. To the extent that beneficiaries use more services such as hospital and physician care than they would if they took appropriate medications, adding drug coverage may help improve the overall delivery of care. It may well lower the health care costs facing society as a result, although expanded coverage under Medicare would certainly mean higher levels of public spending, at least initially. It is always difficult to demonstrate that tacking on a new benefit will not add to costs.

Expanded benefits could be coupled with increased premiums, which probably would result in lower net costs than the current combination of Medicare and Medigap premiums. A key question, however, is whether this should be voluntary or mandatory. A voluntary option for expanded Medicare benefits would tend to attract higher-risk beneficiaries, increasing the premiums that beneficiaries would have to pay. Over time, premiums would continue to rise. An intermediate approach might be to create a two-tiered premium: a mandatory contribution added to Medicare's current Part B premium with modestly expanded benefits and an optional premium covering further benefits to replace Medigap fully. The mandatory premium supplement could be higher than what is needed for a benefit, such as stop-loss protection, in order to help pay for any adverse selection by those who purchase the more expensive package. In the same way that the current, voluntary Part B premium attracts beneficiaries because it is a good deal, participation in an expanded-benefits option needs to attract a large share of the population to avoid risk selection hazards. For example, a subsidy would be required to encourage those who use few drugs at present to enroll. A two-tier approach, moreover, would allow people with employer-provided retiree insurance—who might object to higher premiums for improved benefits they already have—to opt out of the expanded voluntary portion.

The greatest impediment to such a change, however, is the inevitable resistance to higher premiums among beneficiaries and to higher taxes by everyone else.

Further, a two-tier approach may be ineffective in aiding many of the women earlier defined as vulnerable because their incomes often are too high to qualify for low-income protections like Medicaid but too low to be able to absorb readily the larger premiums. If it were tied to improvements in low-income protections, however, women would be better off than under the current system of Medicare plus Medigap on which many of them rely.

The current system still provides grossly inadequate protections for all low-income beneficiaries. Income cutoff levels for eligibility for special benefits offered through Medicaid are restrictive, excluding many modest-income beneficiaries. Limits on what assets can be held also constitute an important Medicaid barrier. Participation in the Medicare savings programs is low, in part because they are housed in the Medicaid program and are therefore "tainted" by association with a welfare program.

For a two-tier system to work, substantial changes in protections for those with low and moderate incomes would be needed. For example, states, which pay part of the costs, are sometimes unenthusiastic about these programs and discourage participation or at least resist efforts to increase it. So beneficiaries alike in all ways except state of residence may face very different levels of protection.

While federalizing this benefit could be expensive, it would raise participation and treat alike people who live in different regions of the country. This is disproportionately of interest to women since they account for 73 percent of beneficiaries with incomes below 150 percent of the poverty level.

OTHER REFORM ISSUES

Although most attention to reform focuses on restructuring options and the benefit package, other significant issues arise, including age of eligibility, beneficiary contributions, the need for more general financing, and improved oversight. Even after accounting for changes that may improve the efficiency of the Medicare program through either structural or incremental reforms, the costs of health care for this population group will still grow as a share of GDP. That will mean that the important issue of who will pay—beneficiaries, taxpayers, or a combination of the two—must ultimately be addressed. These are concerns above and beyond proposals that expand benefits (with the exception of a premium support model, which can be thought of as a financing approach as well as restructuring).

ADDING EDUCATIONAL AND INFORMATIONAL SUPPORT

Considering that Medicare beneficiaries in HMOs tend to have lower education and income levels, the government needs to take a more active role in relaying adequate and understandable information about their options.[10] The state-managed, federally funded information, counseling, and assistance (originally ICA and now SHIP) programs, which are intended to advise beneficiaries about managed care plans and Medicare in general, reach only about 1 percent of Medicare recipients. Most beneficiaries do not know of these programs, and, even if they did, the available resources for counseling activities, many of which rely on volunteers, are so small that only a fraction of people in need of help could be served. Beneficiaries need better education and clearer information about HMOs, their rights as health care consumers in general, and support when they need to appeal wrongful decisions. Women, who more often live alone, can particularly benefit from such aid.

The Bush administration recently advertised its 1-800-Medicare number and beefed up its staffing of that hotline—an important improvement. But it failed to bolster the counseling groups that get the harder questions referred from the 1-800 number. It makes little sense to increase demand for information with insufficient support to back it up.

This help might be further expanded through an ombudsman-type program, providing beneficiaries with enhanced information about their choices between HMOs and other supplemental policies, their rights within HMOs, and the ways to compare different benefit packages, coinsurance, and copayments.[11] Such individuals may be able to reach out to women who are isolated and unaware of possible help. Ombudsmen could help low-income beneficiaries understand Medicaid options. They could sort out eligibility questions, help with applications, and monitor the enrollment process to make sure they receive benefits if they are eligible, again providing a service particularly useful to women. This would build on the SHIP model, which strives for one-on-one counseling. But to be meaningful, many more volunteers for the SHIP hotlines would have to be trained for such work, which would require a substantial infusion of funding. Whether this method or some other approach is used, beneficiaries need considerably greater educational support than they have at present, otherwise, all the discussion about giving beneficiaries choices or empowering consumers means very little. Caregivers, for example, often report that they do not have time to do the research and legwork necessary to find help.

AGE OF ELIGIBILITY

Proposals to raise the age of eligibility for Medicare are offered with the intent to reduce the size of the beneficiary population. Life expectancy has increased by more than three years since Medicare's passage in 1965, offering one justification for delaying eligibility.[12] If people begin to work longer out of choice, delaying their retirement, this option becomes more politically palatable.

About 5 percent of Medicare beneficiaries are age sixty-five and sixty-six. If the age of eligibility were increased to sixty-seven, however, savings would be substantially less—perhaps in the range of 2 to 3 percent of Medicare's overall spending—because younger beneficiaries have lower Medicare costs than others. Also, those age sixty-five and sixty-six who became eligible as disabled beneficiaries would stay on the Medicare roles regardless.[13]

Deferring eligibility has other disadvantages. Without further reforms in the marketplace, those out of the labor force might find it difficult to obtain private insurance. As noted earlier, this matters a great deal for women, who are more likely to be uninsured in their early sixties than are men and would be harmed more by eligibility rising to sixty-seven. Employers will face higher insurance costs if they are compelled to provide retiree benefits to those in their mid-sixties no longer automatically enrolled (yet) in Medicare. Consequently, they might cut back on coverage or become more restrictive in terms of who is eligible for benefits. Extending the time on the job needed to qualify for coverage, for example, is more likely to exclude women.

If the number of uninsured rise—placing further burdens on public hospitals—if the costs of producing goods and services rise in order to pay greater retiree health benefits, if the number of young families supporting their older relatives increase, we will be just as burdened as a society. Although the balance on the federal government's ledgers will improve, we will not have solved anything.

ASKING BENEFICIARIES TO PAY MORE

Some piece of a long-term solution will include increases in contributions from beneficiaries, as it ought to, beyond what was in the Balanced Budget Act. That is, regardless of possible changes to Medicare such as a better benefit package, beneficiaries will be expected to pay a greater share of the costs of current benefits. The question is how to do so fairly. Passing more costs of the program on to beneficiaries needs to be carefully balanced against their ability to absorb these changes (and assessed against other policy changes such as in Social Security).

The easiest way to raise additional revenues from beneficiaries is through an across-the-board increase in the Part B premium. Small percentage increases generate large amounts of resources. The already high cost of care for Medicare beneficiaries suggests caution in this area. And, as a result of earlier policy changes, Medicare beneficiaries will be paying about 12 percent of the total costs of the program by 2008, up from 9 percent in 1998.[14] A higher premium might be more acceptable if combined with an improvement in Medicare benefits.

An alternative, more subtle means of shifting the burden to individuals—often not scrutinized as such—is through a voucher or premium support system. That is, these options can be designed so as to raise premiums for all except a small number of beneficiaries who choose the cheapest plans. While this was discussed above in the context of reducing Medicare's costs through greater efficiency, it also can be considered as a means for increasing the share that beneficiaries pay. The largest premium increases will most likely be incurred by those with the greatest health care needs. If a voucher is constrained to grow at a fixed rate over time, it will probably cover a smaller share of premiums each year. This system would further burden low- and moderate-income beneficiaries who find it difficult to obtain reasonable insurance.

Another option is an income-related premium, for which higher earners pay a greater share of Medicare's costs. This would not place women at a disadvantage because of their typically lower incomes. Tying premiums to income makes sense on grounds of equity, but may be difficult to achieve in practice. Administrative costs would have to rise substantially. But, more important, such approaches fail to generate much new revenue unless the income thresholds at which premiums rise are set very low. For example, the income-related premium proposed by the Senate in 1997, but not enacted, was estimated to have the potential to raise just $1 billion over the period 1998–2002.[15] There simply are not enough high-income elderly people for this option to "solve" the problem without turning it into a welfare program like Medicaid.

ADDITIONAL PUBLIC FINANCING FOR MEDICARE

Ultimately, the issue of who will pay must be resolved by a fair division between beneficiaries and taxpayers. Even with higher beneficiary contributions and more concentrated efforts at improving the efficiency of the program, the long-term costs of Medicare will require additional public funds.[16] Since the population served by Medicare will grow to more than one in every five Americans, as a society we will need to face up to the costs of financing health care, either through the Medicare program or privately.

Reducing Medicare's eligible population or benefits would shrink government liabilities but would do little to change the obligations that society must face over time. For the reasons given here, a public approach to insuring seniors and people with disabilities makes sense. But then we as a society must decide whether to tap payroll taxes, general taxation, or other dedicated revenues. One alternative idea would be to retain the estate tax instead of repealing it. Its revenues could then be dedicated to Medicare. Both tobacco and alcohol taxes have been suggested as potential revenue sources as well. But there is not enough "sin" for such sin taxes to solve the problem on their own. Ultimately the question is one of who should pay and at what point in their lives.

CONCLUSION

What are the appropriate changes to make in Medicare to protect women? First, more attention needs to be paid to the impact of any change on those who are vulnerable because of poor health or low income. Gaps in Medicare have only partially been filled by the Medicaid program. Second, a go-slow approach makes sense when so many of the adjustment mechanisms and other procedures needed to make structural reforms work for beneficiaries are still only crudely developed. Otherwise, reforms threaten to create instability and higher costs for sicker beneficiaries who are not served well by a competitive approach. The information burdens on women as both consumers and caregivers and their higher incidence of chronic illness also make relying on private plans a less attractive option than has often been portrayed. Many women already face the daunting task of enrolling in Medicaid or the Medicare Savings Program to supplement Medicare. And when they live alone, women are less likely to have a support system to help with decisions.

But incremental reforms are not nearly as politically sexy as a major overhaul such as premium support, which may give the latter approach an edge, particularly if it is viewed as postponing hard choices about revenues. Incremental reforms, by contrast, do not allow policymakers the luxury of hoping that the market's magic will provide all the answers from improved benefits to increased cost containment. Thus, some may want to opt for premium support without focusing on its many practical problems. Incremental reforms allow slow and small changes that attempt to balance the program's fiscal health against the health and economic security of its beneficiaries. This cautious approach allows for reconsideration and change if reforms skew too far in one direction or the other. Even with these precautions built in, however, women should beware of changes that represent across-the-board increases in their out-of-pocket costs. But expect the media and political spotlight to be focused more on the flashy approaches than on incrementalism.

Finally, there is much to be said in favor of better coordination of care, even if it comes with certain constraints. For example, a good prescription drug benefit should not encourage overuse of drugs or inappropriate use of brand names when equivalent generic drugs are available. Moreover, even traditional Medicare's methods of operation need to be reconsidered periodically in recognition that more care is not always better. The challenge will be to balance reasonable efforts to hold down costs with evolving precepts of high-quality care.

NOTES

CHAPTER 1

1. Robert Friedland and Laura Summer, *Demography Is Not Destiny* (Washington, D.C.: National Academy on an Aging Society, January 1999).

2. Alexa Hendley, memo, Office of the Deputy Commissioner for Policy, Social Security Administration, February 2, 1999.

3. U.S. Department of Labor, Bureau of Labor Statistics, and U.S. Department of Commerce, Bureau of the Census, *Current Population Survey*, March 2000; authors' calculations.

4. Federal Interagency Forum on Aging-Related Statistics, *Older Americans 2000: Key Indicators of Well-Being* (Washington, D.C.: U.S. Government Printing Office, August 2000). Available online at http://www.agingstats.gov/chartbook2000/OlderAmericans2000.pdf.

5. Joseph Dalaker and Bernadette D. Proctor, "Poverty in the United States: 1999," *Current Population Reports*, Series P60-210, U.S. Department of Commerce, Bureau of the Census, September 2000. Available online at http://www.census.gov/prod/2000pubs/p60-210.pdf.

6. Karen Scott Collins et al., "Health Concerns across a Woman's Lifespan: The Commonwealth Fund 1998 Survey of Women's Health," report no. 332, Commonwealth Fund, New York, May 1999. Available online at http://cmwf.org/programs/ksc_whsurvey99_332.asp.

7. "The Faces of Medicare: Medicare and Women," fact sheet, Henry J. Kaiser Family Foundation, Washington, D.C., 1999. Available online at http://www.kff.org/content/1999/1481/women.pdf.

8. This paper defines persons with physical problems as those who report themselves to be in poor health, who have three or more

serious health conditions, or who are institutionalized. The cognitive measure in Table 1.1 indicates persons with severe mental illness, retardation, or dementia.

9. Linda Fried and Jack M. Guralnik, "Disability in Older Adults: Evidence Regarding Significance, Etiology, and Risk," *Journal of the American Geriatrics Society* 45, no. 1 (January 1997): 92–100.

10. Roger T. Anderson et al., "The Timing of Change: Patterns in Transitions in Functional Status among Elderly Persons," *Journal of Gerontology: Social Sciences* 53B, no. 1 (January 1998): S17–27.

11. Suzanne G. Leveille et al., "Sex Differences in the Prevalence of Mobility Disability in Old Age: The Dynamics of Incidence, Recovery, and Mortality," *Journal of Gerontology: Social Sciences* 55B, no. 1 (January 2000): S41–50.

12. Anderson et al., "Timing of Change."

13. Robyn Stone, Gail Lee Cafferata, and Judith Sangl, "Caregivers of the Frail Elderly: A National Profile," *Gerontologist* 27, no. 5 (October 1987): 616–26; Sheel M. Pandya and Barbara Coleman, "Caregiving and Long-Term Care," Fact Sheet no. FS82, AARP Public Policy Institute, Washington, D.C., December 2000. Available online at http://research.aarp.org/health/fs82_caregiving.html.

14. Frank B. Hobbs and Bonnie L. Damon, "65+ in the United States," U.S. Department of Commerce, Bureau of the Census, *Current Population Reports,* Special Studies, Series P23-190, April 1996. Available online at http://www.census.gov/prod/1/pop/p23–190/p23–190.pdf.

15. Vicki A. Freedman, "Long-Term Admissions to Home Health Agencies: A Life Table Analysis," *Gerontologist* 39, no. 1 (February 1999): 16–24.

16. Anne E. Barrett and Scott M. Lynch, "Caregiving Networks of Elderly Persons: Variation by Marital Status," *Gerontologist* 39, no. 6 (December 1999): 695–704; Jan E. Mutchler and Susan Bullers, "Gender Differences in Formal Care Use in Later Life," *Research on Aging* 16, no. 3 (September 1994): 235–50; Eleanor Palo Stoller and Stephen J. Cutler, "The Impact of Gender on Configurations of Care among Married Couples," *Research on Aging* 14, no. 3 (September 1992): 313–30.

17. Barbara S. Schone and Robin M. Weinick, "Health-Related Behaviors and the Benefits of Marriage for Elderly Persons," *Gerontologist* 38, no. 5 (October 1998): 618–27.

18. Marie R. Haug et al., "Effect of Giving Care on Caregivers' Health," *Research on Aging* 21, no. 4 (July 1999): 515–38.

19. David R. Williams and Chiquita Collins, "U.S. Socioeconomic and Racial Differences in Health:Patterns and Explanations," *Annual Review of Sociology* 21 (1995): 349–86.

20. Catherine C. Boring, Teresa S. Squires, and Tony Tong, "Cancer Statistics, 1992," *CA: A Cancer Journal for Clinicians* 42, no. 1 (January/February 1992): 19–43.

21. Karen Scott Collins et al., "Assessing and Improving Women's Health," in Cynthia Costello and Anne J. Stone, eds., *The American Woman 1994–95: Where We Stand* (New York: W. W. Norton and Co., 1994), pp. 109–53.

22. Williams and Collins, "U.S. Socioeconomic and Racial Differences in Health."

23. "Faces of Medicare."

24. Karen C. Holden and Pamela J. Smock, "The Economic Costs of Marital Dissolution: Why Do Women Bear a Disproportionate Cost?" *Annual Review of Sociology* 17 (1991): 51–78.

25. Jack Fyock et al., "Beneficiary Decisionmaking: The Impact of Labeling Health Plan Choices," *Health Care Financing Review* (Health Care Financing Administration) 23, no. 1 (Fall 2001): 63–75. Available online at http://www.hcfa.gov/pubforms/fyock.pdf.

CHAPTER 2

1. Ronald Andersen, Joanna Lion, and Odin W. Anderson, *Two Decades of Health Services: Social Survey Trends in Use and Expenditure* (Cambridge, Mass.: Ballinger Publishing Company, 1976).

2. Marilyn Moon, *Medicare Now and in the Future*, 2d ed. (Washington, D.C.: Urban Institute, 1996).

3. *Health, United States, 2000 with Adolescent Health Chartbook* (Hyattsville, Md.: National Center for Health Statistics, 2000).

4. Karen Scott Collins et al., "Health Concerns across a Woman's Lifespan: The Commonwealth Fund 1998 Survey of Women's Health," report no. 332, Commonwealth Fund, New York, May 1999. Available online at http://cmwf.org/programs/ksc_whsurvey99_332.asp.

5. Ibid.

6. Madonna Harrington Meyer and Eliza K. Pavalko, "Family, Work, and Access to Health Insurance among Mature Women," *Journal of Health and Social Behavior* 37, no. 4 (December 1996): 311–25.

7. Collins et al., "Health Concerns across a Woman's Lifespan."

8. Deborah J. Chollet and Adele M. Kirk, *Understanding Individual Health Insurance Markets,* Henry J. Kaiser Family Foundation, Washington, D.C., March 1998.

9. *Health, United States, 2000 with Adolescent Health Chartbook.*

10. Marilyn Moon, "Beneath the Averages: An Analysis of Medicare and Private Expenditures," Henry J. Kaiser Family Foundation, Washington, D.C., September 1999. Available online at http://www.kff.org/content/1999/1505/Moonbeneath.pdf.

11. This is different from what many people face in the employer-based system, where choosing a fee-for-service option often means that a higher premium will be required.

12. Out-of-pocket costs comprise all payments made directly by consumers to the providers of health care and the insurance premiums that they pay to cover other health care costs (including Medicare Part B premiums and private supplemental insurance).

13. *2001 Annual Report of the Board of Trustees of the Federal Hospital Insurance Trust Fund* (Washington, D.C.: Government Printing Office, 2001). Available online at http://www.hcfa.gov/pubforms/tr/2002/tr.pdf.

14. *A Profile of Medicare: Chartbook 1998,* Health Care Financing Administration, 1998. Available online at http://www.hcfa.gov/pubforms/chartbk.pdf.

15. *The Implications of Medicare Prescription Drug Proposals for Employers and Retirees,* report prepared by Hewitt Associates LLC for the Henry J. Kaiser Family Foundation, Washington, D.C., July 2000. Available online at http://www.kff.org/content/2000/20000725a/HewittReport.PDF.

16. Stephanie Maxwell, Marilyn Moon, and Misha Segal, "Growth in Medicare and Out-of-Pocket Spending: Impact on Vulnerable Beneficiaries," report no. 430, Commonwealth Fund, New York, January 2001. Available online at http://www.cmwf.org/programs/medfutur/maxwell_increases_430.pdf.

17. Medicare Payment Advisory Commission, *Report to Congress: Medicare Payment Policy,* Washington, D.C., March 2000. Available online at http://www.medpac.gov/publications/congressional_reports/Mar00%20Entire%20report%20.pdf.

18. Marilyn Moon, Niall Brennan, and Misha Segal, "Improving Coverage for Low-Income Medicare Beneficiaries," Policy Brief no. 294, Commonwealth Fund, New York, December 1998. Available online at http://www.cmwf.org/programs/medfutur/moon_improv-coverage_pb_294.asp; U.S. Congress, House, Ways and Means

Committee, *1998 Green Book* (pub. no. WMCP: 105-7), Section 2: Medicare (Washington, D.C.: Government Printing Office, 1998).

19. "A Profile of QMB-Eligible and SLMB-Eligible Medicare Beneficiaries," report prepared by Barents Group LLC for the Health Care Financing Administration, April 7, 1999. Available online at http://www.hcfa.gov/medicaid/dualelig/profile2.pdf.

20. Cathy Schoen et al., "Medicare Beneficiaries: A Population at Risk: Kaiser/Commonwealth Fund 1997 Survey of Medicare Beneficiaries," report no. 308, Henry J. Kaiser Family Foundation, Washington, D.C., and Commonwealth Fund, New York, December 1998. Available online at http://www.cmwf.org/programs/medfutur/medicare_survey97_308.asp.

21. Mark Merlis et al., "Medicare Consumer Information and Risk Selection," Institute for Health Policy Solutions, Washington, D.C., March 27, 1997.

22. "Medicare+Choice: Reforms Have Reduced, but Likely Not Eliminated, Excess Plan Payments," GAO/HEHS-99-144, U.S. General Accounting Office, 1999.

23. "Medicare Reform: Leading Proposals Lay Groundwork, while Design Decisions Lie Ahead," statement of David M. Walker, comptroller general of the United States, before the U.S. Senate, Committee on Finance, GAO/T-HEHS/AIMD-00-103, U.S. General Accounting Office, February 24, 2000. Available online at http://finance.senate.gov/2-24walk.pdf.

24. Jessica Mittler and Marsha Gold, "Medicare+Choice and Medicare Beneficiaries: Monthly Tracking Report for February 2001," no. 25, Mathematica Policy Research, Inc., Washington, D.C., March 7, 2001. A copy can be obtained via e-mail by contacting Lori Achman, Mathematica Policy Research, Inc., lachman@mathematica-mpr.com.

25. Kathryn M. Langwell and Laura A. Esslinger, *Medicare Managed Care: Evidence on Costs, Use, and Quality of Care,* Commonwealth Fund, New York, May 1997. Copies are available from Kathryn M. Langwell, Barents Group LLC, Suite 400, 2001 M Street, N.W., Washington, D.C. 20036.

26. Some individuals maintain plans that they held prior to standardization, and other beneficiaries live in states that specify variations on the standardized plans.

27. Medicare Payment Advisory Commission, *Report to the Congress: Medicare Payment Policy.* For those in the nonstandardized plans, data are less reliable, but many of those beneficiaries do have drug coverage.

28. Lisa Maria B. Alecxih et al., "Key Issues Affecting Accessibility to Medigap Insurance," report no. 243, Commonwealth Fund, New York, August 1997. Executive summary only available online at http://www.cmwf.org/programs/medfutur/alecex.asp.

29. Medicare Payment Advisory Commission, *Report to the Congress: Medicare Payment Policy*.

30. Ibid.

31. *2000 Guide to Health Insurance for People with Medicare*, Health Care Financing Administration, 2000. For ordering information, see the Medigap Compare home page online at http://www.medicare.gov/MGCompare/Home.asp.

32. Alecxih et al., "Key Issues Affecting Consumers' Accessibility to Medigap Insurance."

33. Ibid.

34. Ibid.

35. Judith Feder and Jeanne Lambrew, "Why Medicare Matters to People who Need Long-term Care," *Health Care Financing Review* (Health Care Financing Administration) 18, no. 2 (Winter 1996): 99–112.

36. Carroll L. Estes and James H. Swan, *The Long-Term Care Crisis: Elders Trapped in the No-Care Zone* (Newbury Park, Calif.: Sage Publications, 1993); Penny H. Feldman, Eric Latimer, and Harriet Davidson, "Medicare-funded Home Care for the Frail Elderly and Disabled: Evaluating the Cost Savings and Outcomes of a Service Delivery Reform," *Health Services Research* 31, no. 4 (October 1996): 489–508; Teresa L. Kauf and Ya-Chen Tina Shih, "Use of Home Health Care by ESRD and Medicare Beneficiaries," *Health Care Financing Review* (Health Care Financing Administration) 20, no. 4 (Summer 1999): 127–38.

37. Moon, *Medicare Now and in the Future*.

38. Barbara Gage, "Impact of the BBA on Post-Acute Utilization," *Health Care Financing Review* (Health Care Financing Administration) 20, no. 4 (Summer 1999): 103–25.

39. *Health Care Financing Review: Medicare and Medicaid Statistical Supplement, 1999* (Health Care Financing Administration), 1999.

40. Medicare Payment Advisory Commission, *Report to the Congress: Medicare Payment Policy*.

41. David R. Williams and Chiquita Collins, "U.S. Socioeconomic and Racial Differences in Health: Patterns and Explanations," *Annual Review of Sociology* 21 (1995): 349–86.

42. *Health Care Financing Review: Medicare and Medicaid Statistical Supplement, 1999.*

43. Marian E. Gornick, *Vulnerable Populations and Medicare Services: Why Do Disparities Exist?* (New York: The Century Foundation Press, 2000); Medicare Payment Advisory Commission, *Report to the Congress: Medicare Payment Policy.*

44. John A. Poisal and George S. Chulis, "Medicare Beneficiaries and Drug Coverage," *Health Affairs* 19, no. 2 (March/April 2000): 248–56.

45. Earl P. Steinberg et al., "Beyond Survey Data: A Claims-based Analysis of Drug Use and Spending by the Elderly," *Health Affairs* 19, no. 2 (March/April 2000): 198–211.

46. Jan Blustein, "Drug Coverage and Drug Purchases by Medicare Beneficiaries with Hypertension," *Health Affairs* 19, no. 2 (March/April 2000): 219–30.

47. Poisal and Chulis, "Medicare Beneficiaries and Drug Coverage."

48. Blustein, "Drug Coverage and Drug Purchases by Medicare Beneficiaries with Hypertension."

49. "The Faces of Medicare: Medicare and Women," fact sheet, Henry J. Kaiser Family Foundation, Washington, D.C., 1999. Available online at http://www.kff.org/content/1999/1481/women.pdf.

50. Maxwell, Moon, and Segal, "Growth in Medicare and Out-of-Pocket Spending."

51. Ibid.

52. Patricia B. Nemore, *Variations in State Medicaid Buy-in Practices for Low-Income Medicare Beneficiaries,* Henry J. Kaiser Family Foundation, Washington, D.C., November 1997.

53. "Profile of QMB-Eligible and SLMB-Eligible Medicare Beneficiaries."

54. Richard Kronick and Joy De Beyer, "Risk Adjustment Is Not Enough: Strategies to Limit Risk Selection in the Medicare Program," report no. 240, Commonwealth Fund, New York, August 1997. Executive summary only available online at http://www.cmwf.org/programs/medfutur/kronex.asp.

55. Judith Hibbard and Jacquelyn Jewett, "An Assessment of Medicare Beneficiaries' Understanding of the Differences between the Traditional Medicare Program and HMOs," report no. 9805, AARP Public Policy Institute, Washington, D.C., June 1998. Available online at http://research.aarp.org/health/9805_beneficiaries.pdf.

56. Patricia Neuman et al., "Marketing HMOs to Medicare Beneficiaries," *Health Affairs* 17, no. 4 (July/August 1998): 132–39.

CHAPTER 3

1. Thomas Buchmueller, "Price Sensitivity of Medicare Beneficiaries in a 'Premium Support' Setting," in Marilyn Moon, ed., *Competition with Constraints: Challenges Facing Medicare Reform* (Washington, DC: Urban Institute Press, 2000), pp.135–49.

2. Linda J. Weiss and Jan Blustein, "Faithful Patients: The Effect of Long-Term Physician-Patient Relationships on the Costs and Use of Health Care by Older Americans," *American Journal of Public Health* 86, no. 12 (December 1996): 1742–47.

3. Patricia Neuman et al., "Marketing HMOs to Medicare Beneficiaries," *Health Affairs* 17, no. 4 (July/August 1998): 132–39.

4. Len M. Nichols and Robert D. Reischauer, "Who Really Wants Price Competition in Medicare Managed Care?" *Health Affairs* 19, no. 5 (September/October 2000): 30–43.

5. Sandra Christensen and Judy Shinogle, "Effects of Supplemental Coverage on Use of Services by Medicare Enrollees," *Health Care Financing Review* (Health Care Financing Administration) 19, no. 1 (Fall 1997): 5–17; Stephen T. Parente and William N. Evans, "Effect of Low-Income Elderly Insurance Copayment Subsidies," *Health Care Financing Review* (Health Care Financing Administration) 20, no. 2 (Winter 1998): 19–37.

6. Physician Payment Review Commission (PPRC), *Annual Report to Congress,* 1995.

7. Marsha Gold and Lori Achman, "Trends in Premiums, Cost-Sharing, and Benefits in Medicare+Choice Health Plans, 1999–2001," Issue Brief no. 460, Commonwealth Fund, New York, April 2001. Available online at http://www.cmwf.org/programs/medfutur/gold_trends_ib_460.pdf.

8. Lisa Maria B. Alecxih et al., "Key Issues Affecting Accessibility to Medigap Insurance," report no. 243, Commonwealth Fund, New York, August 1997. Executive summary only available online at http://www.cmwf.org/programs/medfutur/alecex.asp.

9. Michael Gluck and Marilyn Moon, eds., *Financing Medicare's Future: Final Report of the Study Panel on Medicare's Long Term Financing,* National Academy of Social Insurance, Washington, D.C., September 2000.

10. Mark Merlis et al., "Medicare Consumer Information and Risk Selection," Institute for Health Policy Solutions, Washington, D.C., March 27, 1997.

11. Ibid.

12. *Health, United States, 2000 with Adolescent Health Chartbook* (Hyattsville, Md.: National Center for Health Statistics, 2000).

13. Timothy A. Waidmann, "Potential Effects of Raising Medicare's Eligibility Age," *Health Affairs* 17, no. 2 (March/April 1998): 156–64.

14. Stephanie Maxwell, Marilyn Moon, and Misha Segal, "Growth in Medicare and Out-of-Pocket Spending: Impact on Vulnerable Beneficiaries," report no. 430, Commonwealth Fund, New York, January 2001. Available online athttp://www.cmwf.org/programs/medfutur/maxwell_increases_430.pdf.

15. Marilyn Moon, Barbara Gage, and Alison Evans, "An Examination of Key Medicare Provisions in the Balanced Budget Act of 1997," report no. 246, Commonwealth Fund, New York, September1997. Executive summary only available online at http://www.cmwf.org/programs/medfutur/moon246.asp.

16. Gluck and Moon, *Financing Medicare's Future.*

INDEX

Acute care, definition of, 33
Affordability of care: in evaluation of reform proposals, 15, 48–49; problem of, 20
Age of eligibility, proposals to raise, 56–57
Alcohol tax, 59
Arthritis, distribution by gender, 7*f*
Attained age policies, 31

Balanced Budget Act (1997), 13, 26, 29, 40
Beneficiary cost sharing, in Medicare, 24–25; reform proposals and increase in, 57–58; technological developments and increase in, 32. *See also* Out-of-pocket expenses
Benefits, Medicare, 21–23; comprehensiveness of, in evaluation of reform proposals, 15, 47–48; expansion of, proposal for, 46, 54–55
Black women: health status of, 10; poverty among, 10, 11*f*
Blustein, Jan, 35
Bush administration: and information availability on Medicare, 56; and prescription drug coverage proposals, 39

Caregiving, by women, 9–10, 34
Chronic conditions: Medicare benefits for, 2; and out-of-pocket expenses, 36; and prescription drug spending, 34–35; private plans and exclusion of, 45; among women, 4, 6–9, 7*f,* 34
Community-rated premiums, 31
Comprehensiveness of benefits, in evaluation of reform proposals, 15, 47–48
Coordination of care: Medicare and, 45–46; need for, 60; and quality improvements, 50
Costs: health care, increase in, 13; Medicare, by gender, 23*f;* Medicare, by type of service, 22*f;* Medicare, increase in, 13, 40–41; Medicare reform and, 54, 57–58; vs. quality, hard choices about, 49; of supplemental plans, increase in, 52–53. *See also* Beneficiary cost sharing; Out- of-pocket expenses
Counseling, Medicare, 55–56

Disability, among women, 7–8, 8*t*
Divorce: employer-subsidized health insurance after, 19; woman's living standards after, 3

Elderly: share of income spent on health care, 24, 25*f. See also* Women
Eligibility for Medicare, 3, 20, 21; changes in, reform option

ABOUT THE AUTHORS

MARILYN MOON is a Senior Fellow at the Urban Institute in Washington, D.C.

PAMELA HERD is a Robert Wood Johnson Fellow at the University of Michigan—Ann Arbor. She coauthored the first draft of the report with Marilyn Moon.

In addition, Krista Dowling of the Urban Institute provided valuable research assistance for subsequent drafts of the report.

The opinions expressed herein are those of the authors and do not necessarily reflect the views of the officers or trustees of the Urban Institute.